EURHYTHMICS, ART AND EDUCATION

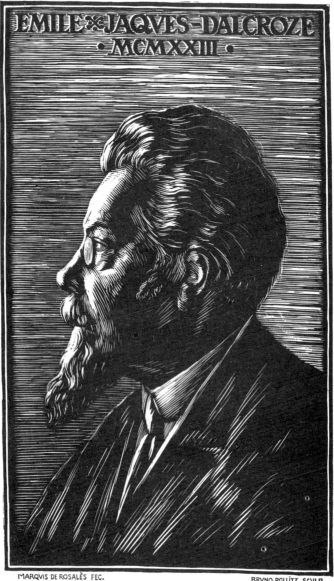

EMILE ✕ JAQUES-DALCROZE
· MCMXXIII ·

MARQVIS DE ROSALÈS FEC.

BRVNO ROLLITZ SCVLP.

EURHYTHMICS
ART AND EDUCATION

E. JAQUES-DALCROZE

TRANSLATED

FROM THE FRENCH BY

FREDERICK ROTHWELL

EDITED AND

PREPARED FOR THE PRESS BY

CYNTHIA COX

ARNO PRESS

A New York Times Company

1976

MT
22
, A74
1976

First published 1930
Reprint Edition 1972 by Benjamin Blom, Inc.
Reprint Edition 1976 by Arno Press Inc.

LC#   78-180027
ISBN: 0-405-08665-2

Manufactured in the United States of America

PREFACE

THE following pages consist of a series of articles written at various times on "Rhythm," *i.e.* the natural force which incites and vivifies, unifies and repeats our acts and wills, the many nuances of which are shaped by circumstances and the demands of our daily tasks, by the unexpected changes of will and the obstacles of all kinds which we meet at every stage of our advance.

Sometimes it is our intellectual processes that modify the natural rhythm of our actions. Or it may be our nervous and muscular inhibitory forces that prevent the complete unfolding of our thoughts.

Is it not the role of the teacher to anticipate in the lives of the little ones whose psycho-physical development is entrusted to him everything that is likely to check the regular evolution of their instincts and their wills? I am certain of one thing: that the rightly-directed will can convert mean and selfish instincts into generous and altruistic ones, negative resolves into positive. The main thing for the educator is to utilise what "is" in building up what may "become": to take advantage of the natural instincts of the children by bringing them under a well-regulated will that is fully aware of the intellectual and physical powers which it has undertaken to bring into harmony.

In order that a race may progress, it is important that there be set up a natural equilibrium between the individual's temperament and his character, and that a sane education of the nervous system promote a fluid and harmonious functioning of all the powers. If the mind is

v

to expand as a whole, it should never be thwarted by the conflicting manifestations of an ill-regulated temperament.

In England for the past twelve years I have had the opportunity of making interesting experiments during my inspection of the schools of Eurhythmics founded and directed by Mr. Percy Ingham, who, at the cost of unremitting effort and by the aid of an admirable organisation, has introduced my method throughout Great Britain and her Dominions and Colonies. Everywhere I have remarked that the metrical side of my system has been very well grasped by almost the whole of the pupils, but the development of the sense of accent and of the powers of imagination still leaves something to be desired, – this being due to a certain lack of excitability of the nerve centres, a certain indolence of the inventive faculties. Thus it is that particular element of education "by rhythm" which consists in rousing the imaginative powers of the human being, that British educationists should consider more especially. They will assuredly attain their object – progress during the past three years is already appreciable – by setting up a constant current between the unconsidered actions of their pupils and their deliberate and co-ordinated acts, strengthening the nervous system by stimuli that call for immediate reactions, and forcing the mind itself to seek personal means of expression by analysing the spontaneous manifestations of the temperament. Thus, in British schools of music, the capacity for hearing is inferior to that of realising music in movement; the rhythmic capacity inferior to the metric. Now, it is my conviction that the British – if musical education in schools be directed towards the quick receptivity of sounds and their immediate and quasi-spontaneous analysis – are destined to become one of the most musical nations in the world, for undoubtedly they are very fond of music – and this is not the case with every country.

Nevertheless, the musicality of a person is always dependent on the possibility of analysing musical acts. It is not enough to vibrate musically in order to be a good musician, for though "life is vibration, vibration is not life."

To return to the standpoint of the physical body, it is not sufficient to cultivate certain motor habits dictated by circumstances, by our environment and mental surroundings, if we would co-operate in this regeneration of the motor instincts which our method of Eurhythmics is an attempt to create. Mind and body, intelligence and instinct, must combine to re-educate and rejuvenate the whole nature. A considerable number of rhythmic currents must establish incessant communication between our powers of realisation and of invention. No enduring progress is possible without the co-operation of a strong and vivid imagination. In these times devoted to sport and to an intensive system of physical culture, it seems to me that we should reflect on the possibilities of setting up relations between our athletic instincts and our cravings for inner harmony. For the human race to be regarded as having definitely reached its goal, it is not sufficient that bodily technique should be taught, in magisterial fashion, by specialists aiming at an impeccable muscular virtuosity. It must likewise be possible for the individual's motor powers – when their collaboration is necessary – to be placed in immediate contact with the cerebral and the emotional faculties, for soul and body to be in mutual and intimate communion, the soul idealising and purifying the body, while the body endows the soul with the strengthening realities of its own energy. . . .

Along such lines may research profitably take place under the ægis of Eurhythmics. The readers of the brief studies brought together in this volume will find a number of suggestions as to the way in which this may be effected.

E. Jaques-Dalcroze

ACKNOWLEDGMENT

THE publishers desire to acknowledge with thanks the courtesy of Messrs. Jobin et Cie, Lausanne, for permission to use the illustrations in this book. These illustrations appear also in various works by the same author, published by Messrs. Jobin et Cie.

CONTENTS

EURHYTHMICS

I

THE NATURE AND VALUE OF RHYTHMIC MOVEMENT

(1922)

THE aim and purpose of all gymnastics is to awaken and develop, by means of repeated exercises, the living mechanism of some particular portion of the human body. Hygienic gymnastics ensures the complete functioning of the body. Athletic gymnastics enables the body to put forth its maximum effort in certain special tests. Vocal gymnastics develops the mechanism of the larynx, the diaphragm, and the lungs, with a view to the effective production of sound. Keyboard gymnastics controls arms, hands, and fingers, enabling them efficiently to interpret pianoforte music.

There is also purely mental gymnastics intended to develop memory, concentration of mind, will, etc. If, therefore, we have to define the rhythmic method of gymnastics, it is an easy matter to affirm that its object is to arouse and develop, by repeated exercises, the natural rhythms of the body. But it will be more difficult to define these rhythms themselves, for they are very complex, or to explain the exercises of the method, for each of them is intended – whether the method demands it or not – to satisfy many different needs. We will at the outset endeavour to explain what are the human rhythms which this method attempts to create and develop.

A rhythm is a series of connected movements forming

a whole and capable of being repeated. The minimum number of movements forming a rhythm is two. The rhythm of breathing consists of inspiration followed by expiration, that of eating consists of absorption followed by deglutition or swallowing. These two elementary rhythms can dispense with education of any kind. Another elementary rhythm, however, that of walking, which also consists of two actions, lightly raising a leg and then placing it heavily on the ground – a rhythm quite natural in the lower animals – requires, in the case of many children, to be called into being by parent or nurse, by means of exercises in passive gymnastics. In other words, this rhythm becomes automatic only after a certain period of training.

Thus we are enabled to affirm the existence of a whole series of human rhythmical actions, which, in order to acquire free, *i.e.* automatic, exercise, cannot dispense with certain preparatory exercises constituting the gymnastics that forms part of all bodily education. Ordinary education, however, makes no attempt to produce more than a few natural rhythms necessary to life, according to modern standards. And when we find ourselves removed from our present conditions of existence and activity, we discover that we are deprived of the use of certain natural rhythms which no longer manifest spontaneously, because they are not directly necessary to our style of life. As a result of the invention of various mechanical modes of locomotion, our legs no longer possess all their original powers of leaping, crawling and climbing. In consequence of our way of clothing ourselves, our feet, elbows, shoulders, and hips have lost somewhat of their suppleness, and oppositions of every kind so violate and warp the mechanism of certain motor habits that combined action – which alone can bring about rhythm – is made difficult, or even impossible.

The gymnastics of hygiene and of athletics restore to the

body a considerable number of natural rhythms which it was thought had been utterly lost, but if we analyse the human organism we see that all its movements do not depend solely on effective muscular action, and that a natural rhythm, expressing some particular state of mind, becomes less regular or free when this mental state is impaired. The spontaneous rhythms of the body have synchronous mental rhythms to collaborate with them. Whenever there is change in a mental rhythm, to restore the balance the bodily rhythm must be modified, and *vice versa*. Unfortunately the balance between the two rhythms is generally compromised by nervous oppositions. The bodily rhythm, thus uninformed, cannot adapt itself to the mental rhythm; the mind combats matter. Hence disorder throughout the organism, disharmony of the various parts of the individual, depriving the psycho-physical faculties of their full freedom of action.

Rhythmic gymnastics attempts to set up relations between instinctive bodily rhythms and those created by the senses or by the will. Rhythm is an indispensable complement both of hygienic and of intellectual or artistic gymnastics.

We are aware that any bad news, any emotion, acts directly on the diaphragm, causing it to contract. So long as the contraction continues, the beating of the heart is modified, the mental rhythms change for the worse, and all active rhythm is hindered. Certain exercises in relaxation enable us rapidly to bring back the diaphragm to its normal state and all our other natural rhythms are released. Equilibrium of organic rhythm depends on the vigour with which we can set at liberty some partial activity whose lack of rhythm compromises the rhythm of the whole. Hence we may well ask ourselves if ordinary education anticipates the possibility of disconnecting the natural rhythms of the child, then of ensuring his reaction to each of them separately, so as to become in a position to harmonise them, even unknown to himself, and to resist instinctively any temporary lack of harmony. This is the problem we are trying to solve.

Certainly we are very far from having attained our object, but the important thing is that a number of teachers and psychologists are now endeavouring to find, in the education of the immediate future, the surest and most rapid means of establishing communication between the various currents of our psycho-physical life and of enabling children's bodies to be under the full control of their thoughts.

Exercises should be threefold: (1) by means of "hopps" – the word of command, coming unexpectedly, conduces to spontaneous bodily rhythms in every part of the body; (2) by repeated appeals to concentration, it lessens the harmful effects of certain ill-timed rhythms and strengthens those of beneficial rhythms, the result being a state of balance between the nerve centres and the muscular forces; (3) by harmonising the functions of the body with those of the mind, it ensures free play and expansion to imagination and feeling through the state of satisfaction and joyful peace that follows.

These exercises should be accompanied by signals or words of command, the object of which is to keep body and mind 'under pressure,' to produce either movements, or sudden halts, or else a combination of halting and moving, to enable the mind to choose from all the muscles the one most necessary for the action demanded and to keep the other muscles motionless; to train the nervous system in such a way that the commands transmitted by the mind may be immediately and completely performed; to combine or to break off imposed rhythms; to combine and interchange spontaneous, *i.e.* involuntary, and reason-

controlled rhythms; to influence the mind by the irresistible might of instinctive rhythmic movements and the
body through the centres of volition; — in a word, to per-
meate the subconscious forces with conscious forces, and
vice versa.

Commands may be given both by sight and by sound,
that is, a direct and immediate imitation or a rapid association of motor ideas in the pupil, is either controlled by the
master's gesture or attitude, or else his *words* influence the
pupil and force him into action. These two sorts of command, however, act only on the will or exercise only reflex
action; consequently they educate only the conscious
powers of the pupils. All that part of education by rhythm
which aims at penetration of the subconscious mind is
entrusted to a more powerful influence than word or sight:
to *music*, a pre-eminently rhythmic art, both exciting and
soothing, which acts not only on the nervous sensibility
but also direct on the feelings.

From its birth, music has registered the rhythms of the
human body of which it is the complete and idealised
sound image. It has been the basis of human emotion all
down the ages. The successive transformations of musical
rhythms, from century to century, correspond so closely
to the transformations of character and temperament that,
if a musical phrase of any typical composition is played,
the entire mental state of the period at which it was composed is revived; and, by association of ideas, there is
aroused within our own bodies the muscular echo or
response of the bodily movements imposed at the period
in question by social conventions and necessities. If we
would restore to the body all the rhythms it has gradually
forgotten, we must not only offer it as models the jolting,
rioting rhythms of savage music, but also gradually
initiate it into the successive transformations which time
has given to these elementary rhythms. Thus, during his

lessons, the master of rhythmic movement must do more than use percussion instruments, like those of negroes or Indians. He will also have to become thoroughly acquainted with the elements of melody and harmony; he must be a musician in the fullest sense of the word.

For rhythmic movement is ennobled by melody and harmony. These rouse the organism, stimulate the muscular energies and strengthen the powers of imagination. Experience has taught us in elementary schools that rhythms *struck* by the master with his hands or by tapping on the ground with a stick can be imitated by the children with considerable accuracy and intelligence, but that they are not encouraged to complete the rhythms or to graduate them for themselves; whereas when played on the piano, there is instilled a spirit of joy and *élan* in both the body and the mind of the little ones, and their powers of invention are directly stimulated. Certainly it is unnecessary that the children should be influenced during a whole lesson by music which deprives them of all freedom of control and makes their task too easy, and so it is better that the music should not be constantly played throughout the lesson or exercises. None the less, it is necessary that the master should have recourse – whenever he wishes – to this higher form of stimulus. Therefore, until man has regained most of his natural rhythms, education by rhythm will need to be supplied by masters who are instinctively musical and acquainted with all the resources of the art. The teacher must know how to use musical methods and employ only music that is simple and appropriate to the age and character of the children.

Some have imagined – the mistake is less common nowadays – that the complexity of these exercises would be calculated to induce a certain amount of brain fatigue in the child. Nothing of the kind ever happens; a state of mental and physical equilibrium cannot possibly create fatigue. It is, however, important that the exercises should be graduated, distributed, and arranged so that the cerebral never predominates over the physical, that each attempt to disconnect or to connect non-spontaneous movements should be preceded by exercises intended to create automatic action, that the child's natural rhythms, from the very outset, should be made so *living* that the constant intervention of new or forgotten rhythms acts as a delightful repose, and, finally, that the master should give at least half the exercises of the lesson in the form of *play*. Under such conditions, there is no need to dread a sense of fatigue. Besides, the master cannot possibly fail to recognise when a child is tired; if inattention or yawning takes place, it is easy to bring about a restful condition either by relaxation exercises or by direct appeals to curiosity or to the imagination.

In connection with relaxation, the beneficent role of exercises intended to check for the moment all nervous, muscular or mental activity is apparently still unknown to many teachers. Exercises in relaxation are particularly useful alike for adolescents and for adults. It would be impossible to insist too strongly on the necessity of making constant comparisons, in the minds of the pupils, between the state of each limb – or of all the limbs – at rest and their different states when active. Besides, it is only through the frequent intervention of a state of complete relaxation that we note the close relations which exist between the muscular gradations of force and the various degrees of duration. In a lesson for adults, one-third of the exercises may be gone through lying down. What a relief when the pupils are then called upon for vigorous spontaneous movements, running and leaping! To my mind it is quite useless to subject amateur pupils to difficult mathematical problems. Is not the main thing, for

adults and children alike, to enable body and mind to interpenetrate? Now, when the mind of an adult is engaged on
the solution of a complicated problem, his body becomes
an inert mass, quite distinct from his mind. To enable the
body to share in the brain activity, the latter must not be
permitted to absorb all the forces of life.

The studies of those engaged in teaching rhythmic
movement must not be applied too vigorously to the solv-
ing of difficult problems. If they would merit the honour
of bringing new principles before future generations, they
should become thoroughly acquainted with these principles and consider every aspect of the problem. At present,
their task is very complex, since the various branches of
rhythmic movement have not yet become specialised. As
a result of this, they have to deal with physiology and
psychology, music and geometry, plastic movement and
education, all at the same time. But the difficulties of this
manifold task need not terrify them. If their knowledge
of music is adequate, and their love for humanity – for
that alone is all-important – strong enough to enable
them to make men's hearts thrill, to instruct and convince
the human mind, they will bring their many and various
labours to a successful issue, for there is one common
element, of singular potency, that animates and unites
them: rhythm.

Musical rhythmic movement consists of linking up
durations, geometry consists of linking up fragments of
space, while living plastic movement links up degrees of
energy. The necessity of undertaking so many different
studies should not appear so difficult that we are afraid to
continue along the path we have mapped out for ourselves.
Think: the small amount of work required to discover the
various mechanical contrivances at the disposal of the
human body involves much investigation and a whole
series of tasks of a different order. Any movement we

have to perform in a given *tempo* requires further muscular preparation if we wish to repeat it in a different *tempo*. A line traversed by a limb in a given space and time becomes shorter or longer according to the degree of energy required to make the movement. A duration of time occupied by a limb moving at a given rate of muscular energy becomes prolonged or shortened according to the length of the space to be traversed.* Moreover, each modification of space, duration, or force, exercises such an influence on the balance of the body that it must be inevitably accompanied by an entire series of correcting efforts made by muscles that either help or hinder. Any error in the transmission of cerebral decisions brings anarchy into the muscular system. All resistance in the nervous system disturbs the brain, and any error of the brain disturbs the nervous system. In a word, the many factors of our life of movement act co-operatively. So also must act the specialised applications of elementary rhythmic movement.

All the laws that govern the harmonising of our bodily rhythms govern that of the specialised rhythms, and set up relations between the arts dealing with sight and those dealing with sound, between architecture and mechanics, between mechanics and music, between music and poetry, between poetry and art, between art and science, between science and life, between life and society. If we are aware that the science of rhythm consists mainly in fixing the laws of balance and economy, and if we make the needed effort to humanise this science in such fashion that we feel it vibrating and thrilling in our own body, as a living part of ourselves, we shall have much less trouble and difficulty in studying its many problems. We shall also expend less time, for we shall be able to economise and balance will and strength, to establish the right relations between strength and time, between time and will.

* See "The Cinema and its Music," p. 208.

Economy and balance: such should be our motto. We must economise our nervous expenditure, which expresses itself in angry starts, sudden, irregular, impatient movements, depression, hypersensitiveness. We must economise our time, cease work before the point of fatigue is reached, anticipate the moment when rest becomes necessary. And we must economise our will to progress, moderate our appetites, and balance our desires of creation with the means at our command.

No doubt at times we have to give ourselves up wholeheartedly in certain directions, to respond to enthusiastic ideals which carry us, as on pinions, beyond the bounds of ordinary life, to powerful impulses and appeals that remove from our minds all petty calculations and prudent self-interests. But we should also be able to recover our balance when this becomes necessary; after wandering astray on the wings of phantasy we must return to the solid realities of existence. From this balancing of our active powers will result greater confidence in ourselves, greater capacity for effectively giving out whatever may be of service to others. It is absolutely necessary that we have confidence both in the end we pursue and in our means of attaining it. Work done in anguish and uncertainty is bad work. From the very beginning we must be able to limit our desire for progress, and not exact from ourselves more than we are able to give out or expend. The one essential point is that we should know clearly what progress Nature enables us to effect, and not stubbornly insist on attempting as much as those who possess greater ability and powers than ourselves. Nor must we forget that inequality in gifts or talents also involves balance: if there were none but superior persons in the world, capable of performing the most complicated educational tasks, there would be no one left to carry out the simple duties of life.

Children need – above all else – masters who love them and make a point of getting to know them. These masters – in the particular case with which we are here dealing – should be able to improvise on the piano correct musical rhythms, they should be acquainted with the mechanism of the body as regards its relations to nervous and cerebral forces, and should also have a certain general culture. In all this, there is nothing beyond human capacity. The one thing to consider before taking up this study is to try to find out how much time and strength it requires, and not obstinately – the only exception to the above-mentioned rule – to attempt to economise this time; for it must not be forgotten that, between action and duration, there exist relations that cannot be modified. . . . If we know all this and do not recoil before difficulties, we shall find that our task is pre-eminently encouraging and productive of happiness; the work of a teacher of rhythmic movement enables him – more than any other person – to react against fatigue and the cares of life. Rhythmic movement is a very focus of energy and joy, and all who study it are upheld by the consciousness that they are aiming at the same goal and are linked to one another by bonds of solid affection which give them renewed strength, security and courage.

II

THE TECHNIQUE OF MOVING PLASTIC
(1922)

THIRTY years ago, there were but few schools that included the culture of the body in their curriculum. Parents were opposed to all gymnastics, and mostly endeavoured to prevent their children from receiving physical instruction, which some of them even regarded as prejudicial to their health! Numerous schoolmasters and doctors condemned the severity of Ling's Swedish drill; the important question of school hygiene did not interest the authorities. The mental outlook has changed since then, open-air exercise has been almost universally adopted, games are played by even the youngest; both at school and at home physical culture is predominant, and teachers and artists alike experience the need of a corporal technique calculated to keep the body in full strength and activity.

Do we mean by this that the many gymnastic systems now in fashion are all equally fitted to prepare the child for a fuller life, to set up close relations between the mechanisms of the body and brain, to unite in one direction the natural rhythms of body and mind? In most of the methods, we do not think that the exercises have any other purpose than to ensure precision and regularity of movement within certain fixed periods of time. They therefore constitute an essentially metrical instruction. In other systems, the spontaneous and instinctive rhythms of the body are the object of closer observation, but the

14

study of the natural relations between muscular dynamism and the laws of agogics or time-divisions – the study of nuances of duration – has not been sufficiently pursued for the pupil to become absolute master of his motor faculties and fit to decide upon the expediency of the movements to be refrained from or of those to be performed. I mean that the body, constantly under pressure, should also be constantly in a state of effortless motion and evolution according to the idea originating in the brain, should react unresistingly to the spontaneous promptings of the fancy; and that, conversely, the instinctive rhythms of a body freed from all intellectual control will enrich the imagination and increase the manifestations both of will and of whim. This technique of reaction as well as of action may be compared with that at the disposal of a fencer, though, instead of being specialised in one or two limbs, it necessitates the co-operation of every part of the body. The acquisition of this technique is the result of a series of extremely complicated actions. Indeed, it takes for granted not only the practical knowledge of all the muscular possibilities of contraction and expansion, in every shade of energy and duration, but also the continual collaboration of the nerve centres, as controlling faculties, with every limb of the body, with each isolated part of that limb, with each association of that limb (or one of its isolated parts) with one or more other parts of the body.

Manifestly, the study of this technique will be facilitated by education in athletics or gymnastics which has previously strengthened and made supple and healthy the organism in question. Nevertheless, the practice of a single sport – or series of sports – specialises the individual in a definite number of movements. On the other hand, the usual gymnastic exercises allow for only a very limited number of variations in speed. Consequently, most athletes or gymnasts employ a certain number of automatic movements prejudicial to the acquiring of that synchronous suppleness of bodily evolutions in time and space which a really complete system of psycho-physical education should exact. They are therefore compelled, when they undertake to introduce art into their motor manifestations, to get rid of certain special technical processes which are too strongly fixed in their muscular memory to allow of variation in the muscular nuances of

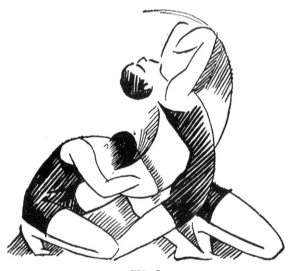

FIG. I

energy and duration. Similarly, in our everyday life, apart from any æsthetic consideration, we feel ourselves checked in motor expansion by habits of poise and gait which constitute the technique of conventional good manners. This technique has been built up throughout the ages by the special conditions of the locality inhabited by man, by his clothing and occupation, by the whole of the social customs and laws which repress his individual temperament. Indeed, the influence of clothes on one's gait is so pronounced that the reproach of walking un-

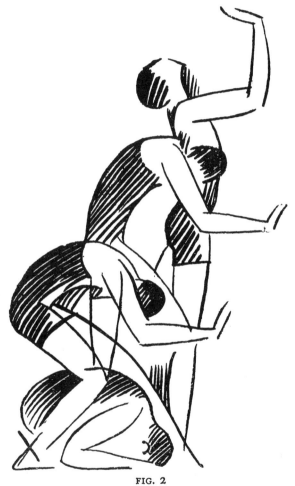

FIG. 2

gracefully in the streets – frequently brought against certain dancers of the modern school – appears to me

c

altogether unjustified. The man who walks naturally and easily in a loose jersey and without footwear, cannot move with ease when wearing tight-fitting clothes and narrow boots with heels.

By what special means can we attempt to restore living or moving plastic, both individual and collective? What new habits of motion are to be created? What fresh combinations are to be sought? What physical means can be placed at the disposal of such technique as will ensure

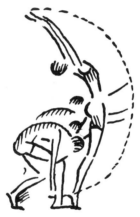

FIG. 3. – Rapid passage from Kneeling to Erect Position

the life and beauty of body movements? These questions we shall endeavour to solve in the following brief account of studies indispensable for our purpose.

1. The study of the means of passing from the state of complete muscular relaxation (recumbent posture) to the various stages of raising the body erect: kneeling, upright position, first without and then with vertical extension of the arms (Fig. 3).

2. The study, when standing, of the effects of breathing on the different parts of the organism, both from the

dynamic and from the spatial point of view; the study also of the relations between the effect of breathing on the expansion and contraction of the limbs in the vocal emission of sound, whether spoken or sung.

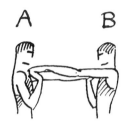

Position at start

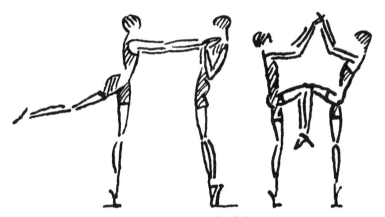

FIG. 4. – Exercises for Balance

3. The study of balance in the upright posture; the points of departure of orientation in the surrounding space, through relaxation of some particular muscular group *; contrasts in weight between differently arranged limbs.

* *E.g.* if a movement to the right is intended, the muscles on the left side will be relaxed, etc.

4. The study of the relations, in the upright posture, between the body and the various divisions of space of which it is the centre. The establishment of distances from centre to periphery. The gradation of space in horizontal, vertical and oblique lines (Figs. 5, 6 and 7).

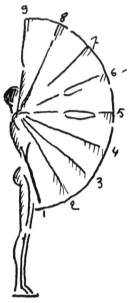

FIG. 5. – The 9 degrees of Orientation in space for Movements of the Arm and Hand

The study of curves. The study of the relations between the amplitude of gestures and the time they take to trace straight or curved lines.

5. The study of the various means of transferring the centre of gravity of the body to another point in space under the impulse of feeling, sensation or will. "Walking" regarded as a succession of divers states of balance, regulated by different intensities of muscular tension and

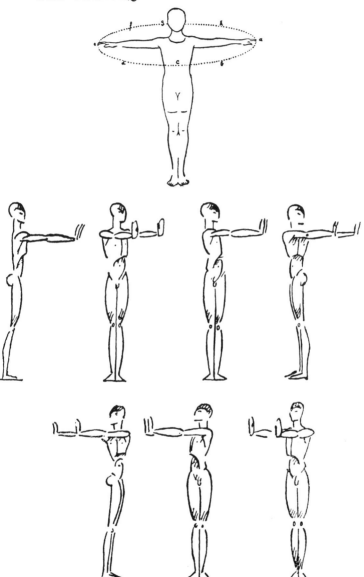

FIG. 6. – Horizontal Movements of Arms in the 8 Segments (par. 4)

different conditions of weight. The various encounters of the ground by foot, leg and foot, body and foot. The body studied in silhouette against walls, or columns, the differ-

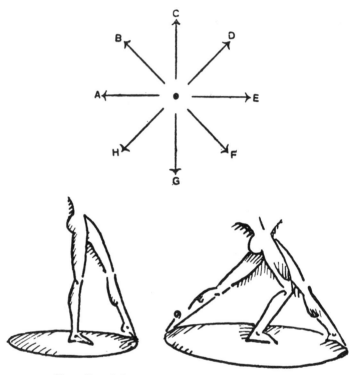

FIG. 7.–Slow Leg Movements (on the spot) in the 8 Horizontal Segments (p. 20, par. 4)

ent height and width of which produce different effects. The study of the several movements of continuous, measured or interrupted progression (Fig. 8).

6. Various durations of measured or continuous steps.

7. Various lengths of step and their relations to dynamics and to duration.

8. The embellishments of progression: running, leaping, skipping, hopping, the alternations of staccato, legato, pizzicato, portando, glissando, etc. (Figs. 9 and 10).

9. Various means of halting in walking, running, leaping, with successions and alternations of these.

10. The study of starting-points in gesture, according as they depend on the displacement of balance of the entire body or on a muscular displacement in some other part of the body or are occasioned by a breathing effect. Differentiation between the gesture caused by yielding to weight and that caused by will to evade weight.

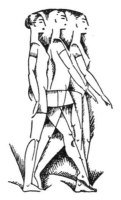

FIG. 8. – Analysis of Slow Transfer of Weight of Body
(p. 20, par. 5)

11. The study of the muscular resistances and oppositions regulating the relations between the gestures of one arm and those of the other or of movements of limbs, shoulders, or bust (Figs. 11, 12 and 19).

12. The influence of bodily attitudes on the material resistances of stage scenery. The collaboration of lines of the body with the lines of partitions, columns, stairs and inclined planes which are made living by contrast.*

* See "*L'œuvre d'art vivant*," by Adolphe Appia (Atar, Geneva).

13. Relations between gesture and walking; their alternation, oppositions, contrasts, agreement and counterpoint. Dissociation and harmonisation of the various motor manifestations of the organism (Fig. 13).

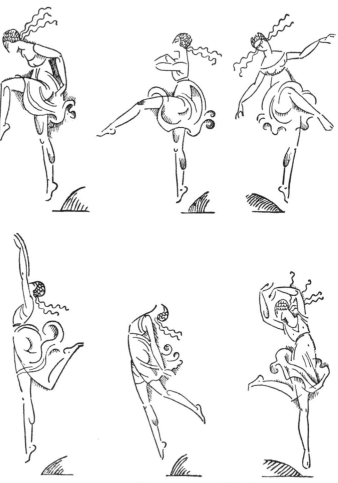

FIG. 9. – Different Ways of Skipping

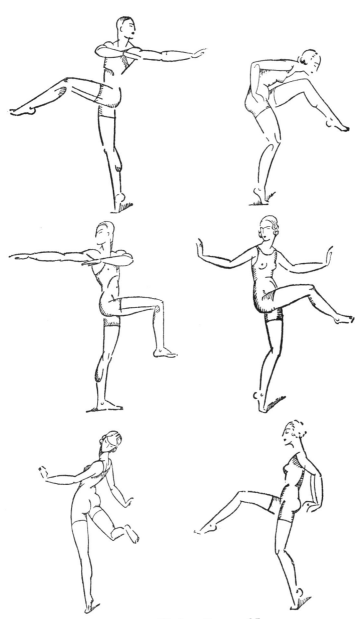

FIG. 10. – Various Forms of Leap

25

14. Relations of the voice (speaking or singing) with walking and gesture.

15. Repetitions of all the above exercises in every degree of energy or duration, one or more limbs twice or thrice as fast or slow. Association and dissociation of durations or dynamisms.

16. The study of the relations between two associated human bodies, harmonisation of their gestures or gait.

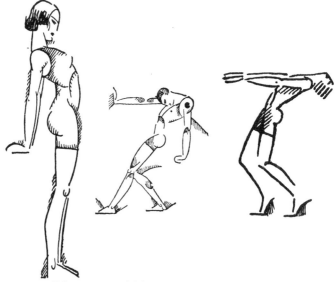

FIG. 11. – Movements of Trunk in opposition to those of Arms
(p. 23, par. 11)

The repose of one individual set against the activity of the other, the opposition of two like or unlike activities both in displacements and in dynamisms at any particular speed (see Figs. 20 and 30, Chap. iv).

17. The study of the relations between associated individuals forming a group, and of the relations between several groupings of individuals, from the threefold point

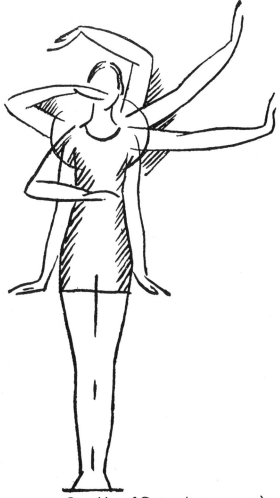

FIG. 12. – Opposition of Gesture (p. 23, par. 11)

of view: division of space, dynamic co-operation and antagonism, gradation of duration (Figs. 15 and 16).

All these studies, however, are no more than the beginnings of the physical technique necessary for a perfect plastic artist. They appeal only to the intellect and the will. The acquisition of all the plastic, dynamic and agogic qualities indispensable to rhythmist or dancer, actor or mime, will make him only an adapter, a trans-

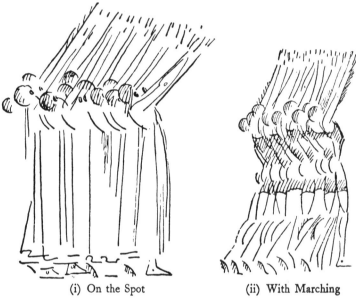

(i) On the Spot   (ii) With Marching

FIG. 13. – Rhythmic Movements of Arms and Trunk (p. 24, par. 13)

poser, an automaton, unless these technical qualities are controlled by wealth of fancy, a supple, elastic temperament, a generous spontaneity of feeling, and an artistic, responsive nature. All plastic education, therefore, should aim especially at the arousing of natural instincts, spontaneity, individual conceptions. The final culmination of studies in moving plastic is certainly the direct expression of æsthetic feelings and emotions without the aid of music

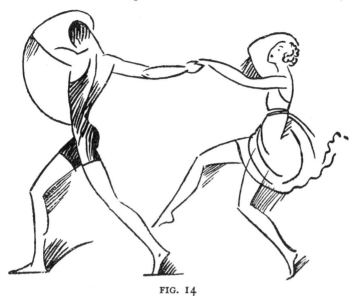

FIG. 14

or even of speech. "Silent" plastic, however, requires wonderful technique gained through an experience that stretches beyond a single human existence. Now, un-

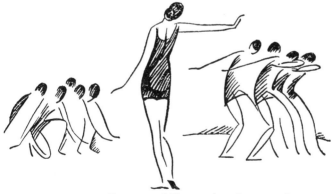

FIG. 15. – Contrast of Groups (p. 26, par. 17)

fortunately, while music is one of the youngest, living plastic may be said to be the least studied, of the arts at the present time. The natural expansions of the body have been thwarted by the habits and customs of a life

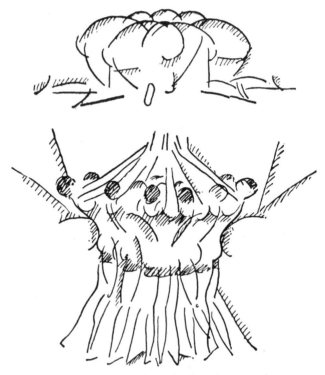

FIG. 16. – Group Exercise (p. 26, par. 17)

increasingly more and more anti-natural. The gamut of gestures and attitudes is thus reduced to the strict minimum. Consequently, the re-education of the corporal means of expression needs support by methods of education adopted from previously tested techniques: those of speech and music. The technique of speech is so highly specialised, and the images it attempts to render concrete follow one another so rapidly, that the movements of the body find some difficulty in harmonising with their form and duration. On the other hand, verbal expression so confuses the realism of the word with the elementary emotion of the thought, that the gesture is constantly wavering between realism and lyricism, between the oratorical and didactic movement and the actual movement. The latter creates the atmosphere and directly expresses emotion by dynamism.

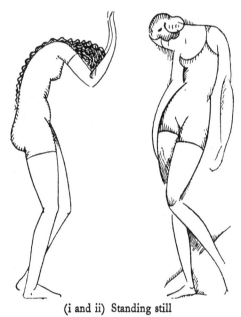

(i and ii) Standing still

FIG. 17. – Exercises in Relaxation

The result is that, while "living plastic" may be allied with words, it is important that, if we desire their full harmonisation, speech should not attempt to remain apart, but on the contrary should ever be thinking of this plastic to which it seeks to become united. That is, the poet should agree to condense his thought into fewer words, to eliminate digressions, to suggest rather than describe, and to regard rests, pauses and suspensions as

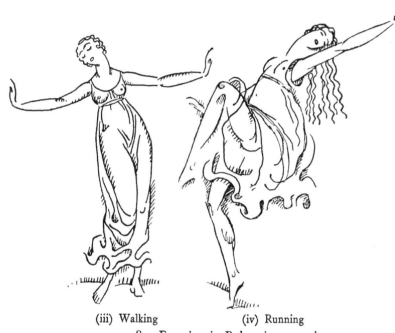

(iii) Walking   (iv) Running

FIG. 18. – Exercises in Relaxation – *contd.*

indispensable collaborators with corporal rhythms; whereas music, which from its very beginning originated in emotion and not in thought, is at present more capable than poetry of intensifying or evoking spontaneous gestures in lyrical situations. It expresses human truths by the aid of sound, dynamic force and duration, in all their gradations. Now, the human body is susceptible of adapting to itself or of transposing the gradations of this dynamic force or those of this duration. But if, disdaining tonal gradations, moving plastic would assert itself apart from them, it will never be able to regulate the gradations of its dynamics and its agogics better than by adopting the musical agogic and dynamic techniques which are now already ordered and regulated and may certainly serve it as models. No doubt living plastic, in its turn, will be able to modify this dynamic and this agogic system, but is not the important thing, in all artistic development, to start with what *is*, if we would reach what may be? And this is so true that even tonal nuance (the varying pitch of sound) is capable, whether in music or in poetic diction, of leading the plastic artist to construct for himself a scale of gestures corresponding to that of sounds. Who knows but that this latter was formerly inspired by the movements of respiration and its action on the muscles of the larynx?

For all who consider the body in motion as a direct interpreter of human emotions, the main thing is to disdain no method of enriching this body's technical means of expression. What matters it if, for some time to come, humanised plastic is allied to music and to words? Is it not important that it should succeed in multiplying and clarifying its means of expression? Now, at such a period as the present, when every effort made tends to link all the arts in one harmonious entente, for the purpose of humanising thought and making it more extensive, diverse and complete, it seems to me that all efforts tending to specialise living plastic would prove barren and likely to lessen its profound importance. As Canudo says: *

* See in the "*Courrier musical*" of April 15, 1921, an article by Canudo on "*La convergence musicale de tous les arts.*"

All energy of impression, representation and evocation of those phalanxes of sensitive beings and creators called "artists," is increasingly influenced by musical laws, by the need of transmitting the most far-reaching laws of life by the help of the most universal of languages, that which "suggests without defining," which alone is able to impose on different collective bodies in varying climates the same ideal emotion. The evolution of music is directly related to the growth of mankind.

The chief peculiarity of music is that it calls forth in the human soul a need for imagination and realisation. Wherefore renounce this power? Music is born within us from the need of escaping from ourselves, of externalising our aspirations, of giving wings to our vague desires, of embodying aspirations that are imperious though frequently indistinct and unco-ordinated. Since it materialises those divine moments when a new being escapes from our usual self, why not place our trust in it, if we would express ourselves by means of a human mechanism as unknown to most human beings as is the origin of their actions and thoughts? To initiate into music artists of the stage and the dance, is to increase their powers, for musical technique will liberate both body and soul.

Is it possible that certain people may not need to study technique because they have an intuitive knowledge of things? Assuredly it is possible. We are all acquainted with child prodigies who play the piano without ever having studied the mechanism of the instrument, young people who are "born" writers or painters, others who dance or act without ever having been taught in any way. Why should it not be possible that certain human bodies may never have known the nervous and muscular, intellectual or moral oppositions so frequently offered to the free course of natural rhythms? Too often the man provided with a faultless motor system is prevented from using it because timidity or lack of self-confidence paralyses his efforts. To be sure of oneself, to be able to forget one's weaknesses, to think solely of the end to be pursued, to feel completely dominated by an idea, is in effect to deny the existence of oppositions; hence, a certain natural technique becomes manifest just when the mind demands it, and that under the excitation of higher emotions. There are certain virtuosi who succeed completely only when they are accompanied by the orchestra, just as there are stammerers who prove to be fluent speakers when compelled to uphold a cause which rouses their enthusiasm. Still, I think that those gifted with this natural technique would be quite wrong not to keep it alive by ordinary regular exercises. Certain stimuli diminish in proportion as age moderates one's spontaneous ardour. A man's progress depends on something more than the ripening of his intellectual powers; each fresh conquest of the spirit needs to be accompanied by improved methods of realisation. The case has frequently been quoted of the Swiss poet, Carl Spitteler, who composed his most inspired poems only after a prolonged struggle to master elementary poetic methods. Verdi, who in the ardour of his youth composed works devoid both of style and ability, deliberately subjected himself to a system of intense musical study which he continued right into old age, in order to produce works of a lasting nature, such as his "Requiem," "Otello," "Falstaff," and his four "pièces sacrées." Chabrier is said to have died in despair at having attempted too late in life to acquire a musical technique with which he had been able to dispense at the outset of his career as a composer. The entire work of Berlioz, pre-eminently a poet-musician, is a revelation of his lack of technical experience, and it would be an easy matter to quote many another creative artist whose decline and fall might be attributed solely to neglect of technical ability. In our present special domain, did we not see the fine artistic efforts of Isadora Duncan, the fervent advocate of natural gesture, checked during the last few years of her life because of a lack of perseverance in acquiring new technical methods? The discoveries of genius need to be supplemented by intelligent investigation. The field of the unconscious, wherein temperament, sensibility and intuition are at work, needs to be enlarged by the acquisition of conscious qualities which enable the temperament first to balance the intellect and then to dominate it without inflicting injury on reason and order.*

And the more the study of certain elementary technical processes of expressive physical technique permeates school instruction, the more easy will it be for the public to understand the efforts of creative artists. The reason why the piano, at the present time, is the most effective means of popularising music is that all our children are more or less acquainted with the technique of the instrument. The teaching of eurhythmics, in the case of children or of amateurs, should guard against excessive specialisation, whether mathematical or metaphysical. At most this teaching will tend to enable pupils to understand the possibilities of the direct relation to metaphysics and to mathematics of the technical education of muscle and nerve which they receive. To be master of one's body, in all its relations with the intellect and with the senses, is to break down the oppositions which paralyse the free development of one's powers of imagination and creation.

As regards the professionals who devote themselves more particularly to plastic study, I am firmly convinced that it is to their advantage to make the organism sensitive by permeating it with music before we allow them to attempt the experiments needed for working out a system to make of living plastic a self-sufficing art, one related in no way to music or poetry. This art will assuredly

* See in *L'Esprit Nouveau*, No. 7, the article by Vincent Huidebro entitled "*La Création pure.*"

appear some day. It will have its own special laws based on geometrical and spatial experiments, their object being to create an architecture in movement, directing and poising itself in accordance with the inevitable influence of a graduated and varied weight. This living architecture will have nothing but rhythm in common with the other arts, but its rhythm will be threefold and will comprise: (1) the knowledge and experience of spontaneous, muscular rhythmic movements; (2) that of rhythmic movements created by modifications of weight; and (3) that of the adaptation of these two rhythms to the unified rhythms of space and duration.

The metaphysics of this integral plastic art will consist in the imagining of fictitious weights and spaces and in modifications and transformations of their relations. Once it succeeds in living its own life, a life governed by laws of its own, plastic art will no longer melt away into music, but will become its ally – as speech is in the lyrical drama. No longer will there be identification, but rather superposition and collaboration. In order to develop, this new art will have to free itself from all direct imitation of nature, all literary preoccupation or mimic intention, and, in my opinion, many and prolonged experiments will be necessary before it sheds all those influences which at present swathe and confine the language of movement. These experiments, it seems to me, must all be of a rhythmic order, and since the natural laws of duration and accentuation of gestures have almost totally disappeared and the number of our spontaneous corporal rhythms is reduced to a strict minimum, I see no other means of reconstituting this new art than by studying rhythm in existing arts, especially in music, which is undoubtedly richer than any other in rhythmic movements.

But we have to consider whether the present is a good time for attempting to construct an integral plastic art.

I am afraid it is not, for this age is keenly bent not so much on specialising its arts as on combining them. The future of art, in the opinion of most present-day artists, lies in the fusion of all the psychic and physical elements of our nature. Never have so many attempts been made at blending together different means of expression. An expressive bodily movement on the stage accompanies sound and words, colour and light. Gifted innovators consider that motion photography will in future be inseparable from a triple symphony; and, not content with dreaming of the synchronism of music and gesture, they attempt to present the moving lines as a series of rigid architectural schemes, and to contrast the rhythms of words and phrases, like the rhythms of thought, with those of vision — to counterpoint, unite and alternate them. They even attempt — in my opinion a mistake — to contrast in the same performance, cinematographic movements with real movements. Certain artist dancers, too, depict landscapes or construct architectural effects by making use of gesture.

The Olympic Games committee, at a meeting in Lausanne, discussed for the first time the proposition of the Baron de Coubertin as to how it might be possible to introduce, in the programme of the fêtes shortly to be held in Paris, human evolutions of an artistic nature combined with appropriate music and scenery. Indeed, the creators of the movement in favour of restoring the Olympic Games have seen that, once education produces men of action, in possession of all their physical and mental powers, there must inevitably be established between them a more powerful bond than the spirit of emulation and the affirmation of self. This bond consists in a common seeking after the eternal laws of art which all have, as their object, to create order, to mould forms, to balance forces and to measure rhythms.

It will evidently be no easy matter to discover how to inspire artistic life in muscular and nervous manifestations that, from the standpoint of sport and hygiene, are self-sufficing. The Greeks supplied us with definite models of gymnastic games, which our own athletes have only to imitate, since the technique of the body cannot be different now from what it was in the time of Pericles. But the evolutions – leaping, walking, running, singing, regulated gymnastic or scenic combats, rhythmic gestures harmonising with the cadences of Greek poetry – were uniformly accompanied by flutes and drums, a music that would not prove acceptable to modern ears. All gymnastic dances and songs in those days were inspired by religious sentiments different from our own. Consequently, it is for us to create new forms of living art dictated by present-day requirements and instincts. Nevertheless, the idea of order in the evolutions, the principle of dynamic accentuation of gestures, step, exclamation and song – all that metro-rhythm which was at the foundation of Grecian artistic manifestations as revealed to us by Pindar, Archilochus and Lucian – should necessarily also inspire the organisers of our modern festivals. Our athletic exercises bring into play three distinct elements: space, time, and dynamics. The relations between them are regulated by the laws of rhythm, and they cannot be distinctively expressed unless those who work them out agree to come under a single control. This latter may be either visual or sonorous, *i.e.* a conductor will insist that bodily rhythms be performed either directly by the aid of gesture, or by means of choral or orchestral music. In the latter case, his gestures will regulate tonal intensity, which will act directly on the ears of the protagonists. In the former, it is his gesture itself that will control the masses.

If we deal with groupings of several thousands of

men, it is easy to understand that an individual gesture cannot exercise its full influence on a number of persons who, as the evolutions take place, are unable to keep their eyes fixed on the co-ordinating element. Nevertheless, if the fêtes took place by night, it would be possible to create a general control of movements, by means of centres of changing light, metrically extinguishing and relighting, the rhythmic coloration of which would act like a conventional orchestra, with a certain definite action upon the masses. Moreover, this method would contribute appreciable æsthetic effects to the *ensemble* of gestures and evolutions. In case the fête took place by day, a display of flags and banners unrolled in every direction and moved up and down, along with "orchestrated" combinations of colours, might be rhythmically arranged either by a conductor or by a machine, in a way sufficiently distinct for the protagonists to obtain the necessary synchronism and polydynamic. These two means of ocular control, however, would lack that propelling, exciting and inciting faculty possessed by music in a higher degree. Naturally, this action-controlling music should be not only understood by the actors but also incorporated in their entire being through the education above mentioned, for our athletic masses will never attain to art unless fresh knowledge is placed within their reach. Art does not spring up by the side of life; it must be born of life itself. Now, the life of our gymnasts is not yet sufficiently imbued with æsthetic sensations for art to be able to appear naturally and spontaneously, as was the case in the glorious Grecian epoch when a knowledge of scanned rhythms, dynamic accentuations and their combinations, was — as Lucian tells us — the foundation of gymnastic and scenic education.

All the masterpieces of Doric sculpture prove the

existence of rhythmic laws which regulate the relations of individuals with one another and the contrasts between various human groupings. All this presupposes on the part of the complete athlete a capacity for adapting himself to every physical rhythm in time and space. Now, in these days, we find many runners who are incapable of performing slow movements; wrestlers who cannot walk lightly; quoit-throwers unable to make any other gesture than that of throwing. Here is the danger of specialisation, a danger incurred by many renowned pianists whose hands and fingers are nimble only when employed on the keyboard!

Sport, I repeat, requires temperament; art requires in addition the sacrifice of certain individual powers to one collective power. The gymnastic exercises of masses of people frequently have extraordinarily powerful æsthetic effects, but they are all effects in simultaneity, whereas the gymnastic art we wish to create needs effects of opposition and contrast, as do all arts.

At a gymnastic fête in Geneva, some years ago, a few thousand gymnasts went through *ensemble* movements to musical accompaniment. The space of ground covered was so extensive that the musical rhythms were some time in reaching the most distant rows, the result being that movements involving bodily displacement, gestures and kneeling, were performed in "canon" style, *i.e.* the first rows kept time, those in the centre were half a second and those farther away a full second later than the first, etc. The result was admirable, and this naturally-regulated polymotivity impressed the spectators far more power-fully than an exact synchronism would have done. It is effects of this kind that the gymnastic art in mass which we wish to create is called on to produce.

To these must be added the effects of contrast which are produced by opposite directions in bodily movement and displacement. Take, for instance, the simple act of kneeling and rising, and suppose that 100 gymnasts are kneeling whilst another 100 are rising: each of the two actions becomes intensified. Suppose, at the same time, that 100 gymnasts raise their arms, 100 others extend them, and that still other rows act simultaneously, some stepping forward, others backward or sideways, and we obtain an idea of spectacles of combined movements very easy to produce. The same in running: if an entire crowd runs, the impression is grandiose; if half the runners stop whilst the rest continue, the effect is doubled. It will be considerably increased if certain runners run twice as fast as the others, if those in certain rows make periodic leaps, if the runners spread out and draw in according to a previously arranged plan.* A game of football (with a real or imaginary ball) arranged so as to obtain decorative groupings and single players crossing one another, will afford the spectators quite a different kind of emotion from that created by a real match. It will not be emotion caused by surprise, but emotion of an æsthetic order, created by the harmonies and counter-points of movements. Doubtless the runners themselves will have less keen sensations than during a real contest, but the sensations will be quite as satisfying, for the joys procured by subordinating the individual to the whole are certainly equivalent to those procured by affirming one's full individuality.

It is difficult to conceive the infinitely diverse possibilities of human groupings. Once an investigation is set up into the effects of contrasts, means of realisation appear and increase. Contrasts of straight and curved lines, of geometrical figures in angles or circles, of different gestures and gaits, contrasts of speed in running, of strength and suppleness of movement, of the number of

* See "The Cinema and its Music," p. 203.

individuals in the formation of groups (groups of eight, of twenty-four, of forty-eight), contrasts with groups of solo performers, of weight and of lightness of step, contrasts of colours and costumes, blues with yellows as a flaring background, and reds drowning greens, contrasts of height, contrasts of sex – teams of men and teams of women – and finally contrasts of opposition between the silence of orchestra and choirs and the activity of human movements, between the repose of bodies perfectly still in various attitudes and tonal dynamisms. We have only to reflect and then will; to imagine and then actualise. Inexhaustible is the mine of contrasts, synergies and antagonisms, of the associations and dissociations of individual and group movements.

Think of the contrast between the various athletic activities, the movements of javelin-throwers combined with running and leaping movements, or contrasted with the movements of throwers of balls. Four hundred men hurl balls into the air, at double or quadruple speed, at different degrees of intensity: a veritable symphony of trajectories. All trades, all bodily activities may be distinctly expressed. The gestures of rowers, of swimmers, of blacksmiths, road-menders, wood-cutters, navvies, mowers and sowers, all supply us with material for distinctive expression. Then, too, the collaboration of the natural human movements with those which necessitate mechanical intervention: ballets of cyclists, the simultaneous evolutions of motor-cars and riders on horseback! Some of these may seem fantastic, though such is not the case: each of these suggestions could easily be put in practice.

So far I have said nothing of the humanisation of the phenomena of nature, i.e. of the imitation, by the body, of the motion of the wind upon fields of corn or waves of the sea, of the placid lines of the horizon, swaying trees, the uneven swirl of a torrent, the wide meanderings of a river, the gushing of a fountain, the incoming tide, the tumultous leaping of flames, or the activity of machines. At each Olympic festival, a general subject might be offered for treatment by human movement, each team being permitted to interpret it after its own fashion. After competitions in strength, suppleness and endurance, wrestling, running and games, there might be held competitions in imagination, organisation and even improvisation.

For there is a new athletic activity to be created: the rapid improvisation of groupings, the arranging and adjusting of this living architecture through the sudden power shown by some imaginative individual over the crowd, or by the intelligent subordination of groupings to the will of one or more controllers. In teaching *ensemble* gymnastic movements, insufficient scope is given for the development of the faculties of imagination and of the spontaneous creation of movements. This may also be affirmed of the cinematograph, whose best group effects are most frequently due to chance, and act on the spectators as picturesque swarmings rather than as æsthetic polyrhythms. Into this domain also it will be necessary to introduce music, though music of a special kind, having nothing in common with pure symphony except rhythm and sound, and, as regards dynamism, obedient to quite new laws. This music will have to be wholly inspired by a knowledge of corporal impulses and muscular rhythms,* as well as of the relations of space with the moving architecture which must occupy it. All attempt at picturesque harmony or counterpoint, all search for interest of timbre, must be subordinated to the physical action, or at least directly inspired by it. More than this, the music we need

* See "The Inner Technique of Rhythm," p. 60, and "Eurhythmics and Art," p. 188. Also "The Cinema and its Music," pp. 195 and 206.

should not constantly accompany the physical manifestations. It should call them forth and sustain them, draw
them out without itself attempting to remain in the fore-
ground. It should also know how to be silent, to oppose
its rhythms to those of the bodily instrument, to counterpoint and unite with them without troubling about any
personal effect. The spectator must forget its very existence, though conscious of its necessity. This music
should originate so directly from corporal rhythms that
the dancers may regard it as the natural expression of their
movements.

Still, even though it be admitted that the art of moving
plastic seeks further means of affirming its existence, and
that, for the time being, it needs the aid of music, it must
not be concluded that music needs to be supplemented by
gesture. Music, indeed, is self-sufficing. Its aim, clearly
defined and attained, is a dual one. On the one hand,
thanks to the Apollonian spirit which inspired it, it frees
us – as Nietzsche practically tells us in his book on the
origin of Greek Tragedy – "from reality by the transfigured representation of appearance." On the other
hand, thanks to the Dionysiac spirit with which it is likewise imbued, it initiates us in the most vivid manner into
the "generating causes of Being and shows us the most
secret bases of things." Simultaneously and successively
it gives form to our dreams and opens out a free path to
our unchained passions. Whether it manifests itself solely
in the Apollonian fashion, as in certain works of Palestrina,
or solely in the Dionysiac fashion as in almost the whole of
Beethoven's work, it still fully expresses "the essence of
dreams and feelings, or that of realities and sensations."
When moving plastic is capable, like music, of expressing
all emotions without the collaboration of another art
whilst giving an impression of order and style, of describ-

ing everything by suggestion, of harmoniously combining external forms whilst revealing the wildest rhythms of
its subconsciousness – then it will live its own life, vibrate
with its own rhythms, assert itself according to its own
ordering. Emancipated from the laws of music, it will
also be emancipated from those of architecture, it will
renounce mimicry – a process accessory to imitation – it
will have its own style, its forms and nuances, and we shall
realise that Pasmanik is right in affirming "that no art
requires collaboration from without, and that no sooner
does it become incarnate in a perfect product than it suggests, by its own inherent power, all the effects the other
arts are capable of producing."

When, however, each of the arts becomes autodynamic
and autonomous, none of them will be constrained to
maintain for ever a splendid isolation. There will still
have to be created the laws of a universal harmony,
dictating for each specialised art what sacrifices and
eliminations will be necessary for effective collaboration.
And then, by means of these eliminations, each of the arts,
without losing its own personality, may be called upon to
supplement a sister art, which for the time being has
voluntarily decided not to be constantly using all its
means of expression. And in certain circumstances we
shall find all the arts blending in one grand symphony.
There will appear works in which moving plastic, for
instance, will constitute the element of order; music, the
element of emotion; words, the element of dreamland . . .
and *vice versa*. All combinations will become possible,
and discussion as to the expediency of a fusion of all
æsthetic elements will become futile. The reason why so
many artists discuss this subject nowadays – and frequently with so much feeling – is that these elements have
not yet been distinctly classified, or even established. It is
a matter of importance that all arists, now striving to

effect a renaissance of the great popular spectacles based
on the art of movement, should frankly impart to one
another their experiences and discoveries, and, without
vainly setting up one art against another, appreciate
beauty and truth in whatsoever guise. Thus will they
contribute not only to their own happiness but also to the
happiness of the various peoples and races and to the
general progress of mankind.

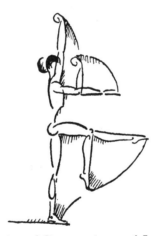

FIG. 19. – Association of Gesture: Arm and Leg (p. 23, par. 11)

III

THE INNER TECHNIQUE OF RHYTHM
(1925)

Iᴛ is but little more than a century since music ceased to be an art cultivated by a few privileged individuals, to become an essentially popular art taught from childhood to almost the whole of mankind, without thought of natural talent or exceptional ability. Music schools once frequented solely by highly-gifted musicians now welcome all who love music, even though they lack the indispensable capacities for musical expression and execution. The number of brilliant pianists and violinists daily increases, everywhere instrumental technique makes amazing progress, but observers wonder whether the quality of the instrumentalists is equal to the quantity, whether the acquisition of an extraordinary technique is calculated to further the cause of music unless this technique be combined with musical ability which, if not first-class, is at least normal.

Formerly, instrumentalists without exception were fully-equipped musicians, all of them capable of improvising and composing, artists irresistibly attracted to art by a noble urge toward æsthetic emotion, whereas the majority of young people who now aspire to excellence are content to imitate the emotion of the composer without being capable of experiencing it themselves, and possess no sensibility but that of the fingers, no originality but that of their masters, no executive ability but a painfully acquired automatism. The musical virtuosity of the present day is too often specialised in a finger technique which is quite distinct from the intellectual and emotional faculties and shows itself only in speed passages. Technique is no longer a means; it has become an end.

A programme of musical studies nowadays is not what it ought to be; it would be impossible for a pupil to become a musician by means of these studies if he were not already one before he began them. Consequently, musical studies are now illogical and incomplete, as it is taken for granted that they must be followed by *gifted* individuals, whereas too frequently they are followed by music lovers, of the utmost good will doubtless, but on whom nature has but imperfectly lavished the physiological faculties needed by the musician. These qualities are delicacy of aural perception, nervous sensibility, rhythmic feeling, *i.e.* the true sense of the relations between movements in time and those in space – and, lastly, the faculty of spontaneously externalising sensations of movement and transforming them into feelings and emotions – *i.e.* the imaginative and creative sense.

Delicacy of aural perception enables the musician to acquire a knowledge of every variety and shade of sound combinations; nervous sensibility makes it possible for him to experience and recognise all shades of sensation; rhythmic feeling enables him to experience and recognise all distinctions of speed and dynamics. Lastly, the power to transform sensations into feelings, and conversely to express emotions plastically, enables him immediately to give effect to his imaginative conceptions, to set up a current between his intellectual and his physical faculties, between his muscular organism and his artistic fancies. It is only when all these various qualities are found, even if in embryo, in the future musician, that musical studies can make a true artist of him; for they prove that music *is in him*, forms part of his being, and will grow by the exercise of these faculties. But if they are non-existent, how can instrumental studies be expected to develop them? And how can the future musician help becoming a mere imitator, a spectator of art, instead of being a recipient and a transformer of artistic sensations?

All modern schoolmasters agree that the child's first education consists in teaching him to know himself, in familiarising him with life, and arousing in him sensations, feelings and emotions before enabling him to describe them. In modern schools of art the pupil is taught *to see* the things before he paints them. In music, unfortunately, this is not the case; children are taught to play Bach, Mozart, Beethoven, Chopin, Liszt, and Debussy, before their minds and ears are open to the understanding of these works, before their bodies have developed the power of being moved by them. Now, does not such a mode of education seem calculated to do a great deal of harm to the art of music itself, and also to cause in the individual practising it a certain loss of time and strength, a diminishing of his personality? *

During the twenty years I have been professor of harmony at the Conservatoire of Geneva, I have had many opportunities of recognising how defective in the most elementary musical ability were the majority of my pupils, even the most advanced. I found the simplest elements – the recognition of pitch and the sense of rhythm – so imperfectly developed that theoretical teaching could be given only in the most tortuous way and through continual obstacles. It was through discovering that nine out of every ten pupils understand and "live" music so little that I resolved to give all my time to the development of the child's musical powers, so that he might subsequently be passed on to his instrumental and technical studies under conditions which would enable him to regard this

* See "The Piano and Musicianship," Chap. VII.

very technique as a means of asserting himself, of carrying out his personal determination and feelings, instead of allowing it to become a means of slavishly imitating the thoughts and feelings of others.

There are two physical agencies through which we appreciate and understand, live and experience music: the ear, as regards sound; the entire nervous system, as regards rhythm. Experience proves that it is not easy to educate both of these simultaneously. A child finds it difficult to apprehend a melodic succession and the rhythm animating it at the same time. Before teaching the relations between sound and movement, it is wise to study these two elements separately. Sound is manifestly of secondary importance since it has not its origin and model within ourselves; whereas movement is instinctive in man, and therefore first in importance. And so I begin musical studies by the methodical and experimental teaching of movement.

There are two kinds of movement: spontaneous and deliberate. The former depends on the temperament and creates rhythms; the latter depends on the character and creates measure. Certain children have neither muscular nor nervous oppositions, they measure their movements without having been taught. These children are not necessarily rhythmical; they very frequently lack those spontaneous impulses, those alternations of opposition and surrender, rigidity and suppleness, elasticity and firmness which produce rhythm. The first thing to teach such children is a greater capacity for vibration. Special exercises will attempt to arouse and then stimulate their nervous sensibility, to develop their reactions, to increase the number of their movements. Other children are of a very lively temperament; they react rapidly to the word of command, their impulses are spontaneous and irresistible, but they cannot regulate their movements, harmonise their instincts. Such children from the very beginning should be given exercises in metre; they should be taught to introduce order into their vital manifestations.

The metric exercises will first be marching exercises, for walking is the natural model of time. The various musical bar-times will be taught by accentuations of the foot; pauses of various lengths will teach the children to differentiate between the note-values (minim, dotted minim, semibreve, etc.); measured gestures of arms and head will maintain order in the succession of note-values and will analyse bar-times and duration of sounds; regular breathing will introduce the study of phrasing, and exercises in the crescendo and the decrescendo of muscular innervation will introduce that of nuance. Perhaps the reader thinks all this quite simple to put in practice, and so I thought at the beginning of my experiments. These, unfortunately, have shown me that the matter is very complicated. Why is this? Because Nature has created extraordinarily different types and has established innumerable shades of character. There are children who possess the instinct of time but not that of accentuation, and *vice versa;* the movements of others are harmonious, but they have no idea of balance. Others again at once understand a rhythm, but are unable to continue it without modifying it, etc., etc. Powers of motion are not alike in all men; there are many hindrances to the exact and rapid physical expression of mental conceptions. In stepping, one child is always behind, another always in front; one advances with unequal steps, another is incapable of taking a single irregular step, even exceptionally.* If these defects are not corrected in the early years, they will subsequently appear in the playing of music. Singing or playing too fast or too slow, a "stammering"

* See "General Education and Rhythmic Movement," p. 103.

performance, inability to accompany a singer or an instrumentalist, over-harsh or too indefinite accentuation, etc. — all these are due to a lack of correlation between the mind which conceives the movement, the brain which orders it, the nerve which transmits the order and the muscle which executes it. Again, the power to phrase and shade music correctly and artistically depends alike on education of the nerve centres, harmonisation of the muscular system, and rapid communication between limbs and brain; in a word, on the health of the entire organism.

It was by endeavouring to determine the individual cause of each musical defect and to find a remedy for it that I gradually built up my method of rhythmic gymnastics. This is based entirely on repeated experiments, and not one of these exercises has been adopted or written down until it has been applied in many forms and under various conditions, and its utility seemed to me indisputably proved. An art critic recently published in a Paris magazine an article in which he took me to task for my methods of giving the word of command. He criticised the "imperative hopps" intended to create sudden reactions in the pupil. In thus blaming me, does he not give evidence of the inadequacy of his own hearing — a pardonable fault — to grasp the many dynamic varieties of these "hopps"? Of course it is indispensable, in stimulating an energetic reaction in pupils with sluggish nervous systems, to have recourse to sharp words of command. But the "hopps" vary in intensity according to the nature of the reactions desired. During the first year's instruction, they are given two, three, four beats in advance; at the completion of the course, the master utters the word half a second before it is carried out. The "hopp" is frequently replaced by a sign of the hand, an interruption or a musical change in the playing of the piano. It is actually this variety of command that ensures for the pupils the true development of their personality, and all teachers who have conscientiously followed these experiments know how different they are from the usual drill exercises. Moreover, it is very difficult to judge of new exercises in education without going through them oneself, and rhythmic gymnastics is above all else *personal*. It aims at creating, by rhythm, a stream of rapid and regular communication between brain and body. The thing that completely differentiates these physical exercises from those of the usual methods of muscular development is that each exercise is conceived in the form which has to set up most rapidly – and to fix definitely in the brain – the image of the movement studied In all muscular action, the untimely intervention of useless muscles has to be voluntarily eliminated, so as to develop attention and will, and then an automatic technique to be created for all muscular movements which do not need the aid of attention, so that this latter way may be reserved for the purely intelligent manifestations of the individual.

Rhythm is an element of an irrational nature. Metre exists and is maintained only through reasoning: it develops the powers of control. To vibrate *without metre*, then to express oneself *in metre*: such is the province of man and of the perfect artist. From the very fact that rhythm harmonises the nervous centres and creates a greater possible number of motor habits, education based on an experience of rhythm evokes and ensures freedom for the greatest number of subconscious manifestations, and those, instead of manifesting themselves wildly, losing half their force because they cannot be concentrated in one direction, will profit by the order and harmony set up in the organism, combine with the conscious powers of the individual and ensure his all-round development.

Wild-flowers grow in greater abundance and beauty in a well-tilled garden than in a state of nature, where most of them are overrun with brambles or fade away in the shade. The creation in the human body of a rapid and light system of communication, between all the agents of movement and thought, gives free and untrammelled action to the personality; it strengthens and vivifies this personality in the most amazing way. It also gives the individual the self-confidence necessary for well-balanced vital functions, since it enables him easily to give effect to each of his conceptions. Frequently neurasthenia is nothing but an intellectual disorder produced by the incapacity of the nervous system to obtain from the muscular system a regular obedience to cerebral orders. It is the education of the nerve centres, the establishment of order in the body which is the sole remedy against intellectual perversion – the product of lack of will and of the incomplete subjection of the body to the commands of the mind. Incapable of realising its conceptions materially, the brain amuses itself in creating images without any hope of giving effect to them, it drops the substance for the shadow, and substitutes vague and empty mental speculations for the free and healthy union of mind and matter.

If we adopt the artistic point of view, by placing the fully developed faculties of the individual at the service of art, this education gives it the most perfect and supple of interpreters, the human body, which may become a marvellous instrument of beauty and harmony when attuned to the artistic imagination and collaborating with creative thought. It is not enough that music pupils, by means of special exercises, should have corrected their faults and no longer risk compromising their musical interpretations by ungainly limbs and disharmonious movements; the music which *has its abode in them* – artists will understand me – must be capable of free and entire development and the rhythms that inspire their natural emotions must enter into close communion with those that inspire the works to be interpreted. The nervous system must be so educated that the rhythms suggestive of the work of art may call forth similar vibrations in the individual, produce a powerful reaction, and become quite naturally transformed into actual rhythms. Similarly, in pictorial, architectural and sculptural art it is not enough to have schools for teaching the representation of lines and colours, lights and shades, reliefs and massed groups: the pupils must learn to feel within themselves the rhythmic movement which balances, harmonises and animates a work of art. In simpler language, the body must become susceptible of emotion under the influence of artistic rhythms and give effect to them quite naturally, without either timidity or exaggeration. This faculty of emotion, indispensable to the artist, was – as I said at the outset – natural in the past to almost all who were learning music, for there were scarcely any but born artists who gave themselves up to music; but I maintain that, while such is not the general rule nowadays, it is at all events possible to arouse latent faculties, to develop and harmonise them, and that every music teacher is in duty bound to deter from instrumental technique anyone lacking in musical feeling and incapable of responding to artistic emotion. It is rhythm that sets up communication between our inner forces and the outer forces that assail them. The experimental study of rhythm should form part of all well-organised musical education.

This study will prove beneficial to music itself, as well as to musicians. In proportion as new harmonic and orchestral methods have been framed and practised, it has been the aim of musical instruction to enable the coming musicians to benefit by the progress attained by modern composers. Treatises on harmony and instrumentation deal with new acquisitions; theoretical teaching facilitates their diffusion. The same cannot be said of discoveries in the world of rhythm during the past twenty years. Not one book on musical theory out of four even mentions them, and the imaginative process which impelled such men as Brahms, Ravel, Stravinsky, Schönberg, Holst, etc., to bring forth full-fledged, richer, more original and complex rhythms, is only occasionally analysed by the theorists. The music student should divine and formulate for himself the laws governing composition and the inter-weaving of new rhythms. Wise teaching should help him to acquire this new technique; it is to be regretted that such instruction so seldom exists in many professional schools of music. Rhythmic experiments, a complete study of movements and their combinations, should create a new mental attitude. Under this training artists will spontaneously and inevitably invent new rhythmic forms to express their feelings; consequently their personality will find an opportunity for more complete self-development, for more powerful self-assertion. Musical children, subjected during the requisite period of time to an education by rhythm, quite naturally imagine original rhythms which might never enter the head of a professional musician; they will find monotonous many contemporary works which are poor in rhythm, though rich in harmony and instrumental effects.

I have said that rhythmic gymnastics – whatever method of teaching may be adopted – is more than an educational method. Indeed, it is a force analogous to electricity and the great natural forces of chemistry and physics; it is an energy, a radio-active agent whose influence restores us to ourselves, in making us aware, not only of our own powers, but also of those of others, those of humanity. It compels us to meditate upon the unfathomable depths of our enigmatical and changing nature. It enables us to glimpse the secrets of the eternal mystery which governs the lives of men throughout the ages, it gives our thoughts that original character of intense religious feeling which links together the past, the present, and the future, to create closer relations between body and mind, to unify the moral and physical forces of the individual, and to give a firmer foundation to the relations between men.

The object of education is to enable pupils to say at the end of their studies, not 'I know,' but 'I experience,' and then to create the desire of *self-expression*. For when we experience an emotion strongly, we feel the need to pass it on to others, to the utmost of our power. The more life we have, the more we shall be able to give to others. To receive and to give: such is the great rule for all mankind. The reason why I construct my entire system upon music is because music is a great psychic force, a resultant of our functions of mind and expression which, through its power of stimulation and regularisation can bring order into all our vital functions.

Creative of order, music, more than all other arts, is able to manifest in time all the various shades of our feelings. Every man should have *music within himself*. I mean what the Greeks called music, *i.e.* the totality of our sensorial and psychic faculties, the ever-changing symphony of spontaneous feelings created, modified, then refined by the imagination, ordered by rhythm and harmonised by consciousness.

No observing artist can deny that a conscientious study of rhythm in all its forms may bring the pupil to a more living understanding of art. Art consists alike of imagination, reflection and emotion. Reflection tempers and refines imagination. Imagination animates and vivifies style. Emotion ennobles and makes apparent the results of reflection and imagination.

The object of art studies is not solely to educate artists capable of communicating æsthetic impressions to the public; they also aim at forming a public able to appreciate the artistic representations offered to it, to unite with them and be vividly conscious of the emotions manifested in them. School instruction is not enough; the education of mind and senses has for its mission to raise the public to such a level that it may become a true collaborator in the symbolic and poetical spectacles which the most gifted men are capable of offering it. An education in rhythm is capable of arousing the artistic sense.

A true teacher should be both psychologist, physiologist, and artist. When a pupil leaves school, he should be capable not only of living normally but also of feeling life with a certain emotion. He should be put in a position to create, to thrill in accord with the emotions of others. Only an artistic education, entering largely into physical exercise, can bring calm to an over-excited nervous system. If this education is essentially of the nature of sport, it will outstrip its object and produce generations devoid of sensibility. It is important that education should devote like attention to intellectual and to physical development, and as rhythmic gymnastics possesses this dual qualification, its influence must be a beneficent one.

I cannot conclude this brief exposition without mentioning the close relations between movements in time and those in space, between sound-rhythms and body-rhythms, between music and plastic. Gestures and attitudes complete, animate and vivify all rhythmic music simply and naturally conceived without any exclusive concern for sound. As in painting there exist side by side a school for the nude and one for landscape, so there may develop side by side 'plastic' music and 'pure' music. In the landscape school, emotion is created by line movement animated by the many combinations of light and the rhythms which light sets vibrating in everything that comes under its sway. The effect is not produced by the landscape itself but by the emotion born of illumination in the soul of the painter. In the school of the nude, showing the many shades of expression of the human body, the artist subordinates his own emotion to that of the human subject to be depicted. He endeavours to show as he imagines it to himself the soul of man modelled by the body forms, coloured by the emotion of the moment. At the same time, he depicts the essential character of the individual and the race, asserting himself through the modifications of equilibrium imposed by the temporary emotional state. . . . Similarly pure music, in its construction and its melodic and harmonic developments, will reveal the very soul of the creative artist, whilst he will attempt in plastic music to depict the feelings of humanity as revealed to him in gesture and attitude. He will model sounds after rhythmic forms created direct by the expressions of the human body, or rather, will suggest to this body rhythms susceptible of being transposed direct from the domain of sound to that of plastic. The rhythms of plastic music take as models those created by the nervous and muscular systems. To compose that music – which the Greeks appear to have realised and which Goethe and Schiller subsequently divined – it is absolutely necessary that musicians have personal experience of body movements and of their relation to the life of emotion, while interpreters will naturally have to be subject to a similar education.* They have no need, in plastic interpretation, to make visible all the details of musical rhythms, but to become imbued with their character and to share wholeheartedly in their impulses.

* See "The Technique of Moving Plastic," p. 44. Also "Eurhythmics and Art," p. 188; also "The Cinema and its Music," pp. 195 and 206.

A rational and conscious plastic interpretation of musical rhythms is based wholly on pantomime. In the lyric domain, on the other hand, we are dealing with a quite distinctive transformation of sound movement into body movement by means of an intimate permeation of the emotional essence of music. The classic unity of the dramatic musical product, the fusion of gesture, music and word, is at present realised only in exceptional cases, for though music and word, though word and gesture, are closely blended in certain works, it is far more rare to find communion between gesture and music. In the majority of singers, this communion can be effected only by special education. Man will thus regain his natural means of expression along with all his powers of movement, and art has everything to expect from new generations brought up in the cults or orderliness and truth, of physical and moral harmony and health.

It is by a voluntary reversion to simplicity, to freedom of expression, to a natural abandonment of the entire being to artistic emotion, that — apart from all intellectual picturesqueness — the musico-plastic art of the immediate future will grow and develop. The artist must spiritualise himself before desiring or being able to spiritualise matter. Art should be expressive in essence and potency, not imitative or impressionist. Plato said: "Beauty is the splendour of Truth," and Goethe added: "In plastic and musical art lie hid the profoundest secrets of human sensibility."

IV

PHYSICAL TECHNIQUE AND CONTINUOUS MOVEMENTS

PHYSICAL technique practised for an artistic end ought to develop a combination of qualities which should enable men to give expression to every shade of thought and emotion by means of the resources of the body. But many still consider that physical training aims, as well as this, at out-doing nature, and enabling one to excel in exercises of speed, balance, and leaping; if a man does not become a brilliant virtuoso, the training is considered imperfect. Similarly, to a certain type of musical critic, a pianist with complete control of his nervous impulses, a sensitive touch and a delicate sense of rhythm, phrasing, and accentuation, will nevertheless only be considered to possess a fine technique if these qualities are displayed at express speed. On the other hand, if he can perform passages of transcendent virtuosity, his technique will be considered good, even though he lack the musical attributes described.

In reality there are many kinds of technique. The Cambodian and Javanese dancers have a highly-developed technique of the arms, hands and fingers, but not that of walking, running, or leaping. They would be unable to attempt the Icarian leaps of the Russians; but, incapable of rapid movements, prefer to remain faithful to their favourite bent-leg attitudes. Should such dancers, although they lack the technique of the leap, be qualified as poor exponents of bodily movement and living plastic?

On the other hand, many dancers who excel in toe-work and gyrations and who possess all the physical resources developed through classical dancing, cannot walk naturally and are singularly deficient in power of expression by means of the hands, wrists, arms, and trunk. Simply a different technique.

The negroes possess extraordinary dexterity of thigh, knee and foot, and their speciality is the bending and twisting of the lower parts of the body. Are we to say they lack technique because of the almost pathetic stupidity of their unexpressive, relaxed arms and shoulders?

Amusing errors are committed by critics and writers on dancing and bodily expression. It can scarcely be expected that a clarinettist should possess the same technique as a violinist, or a 'cellist that of a tuba-player; and if the human body is regarded as an instrument, it must not be concluded that the instrument is the same in all men. One may be a born jumper, another may excel in running, a third may instinctively possess a knowledge of expressive arm-gestures and attitudes. All dancers can acquire by study the elementary qualities of balance, natural movement and harmony of gesture, but it is rare that the whole of its motor faculties can be obtained from the human body. Just as a tenor would cut a sorry figure if required to sing a bass part, so would an "all-round athlete" figure poorly in a choreographic interlude.

Certainly a good dancer ought to have a knowledge of all styles and be prepared to interpret all kinds of music. There are some who possess the necessary physical suppleness to accomplish this, but are handicapped by lack of suppleness of mind and imagination and by knowing nothing of dynamic and agogic shading. This is because in classical dance-training nothing is addressed to the mind, the taste or the fancy, or to the sense of proportion,

phrasing and expression. The same automatic movements are employed for all interpretation; the same types
of leaps, turns and pirouettes are found in the most
diverse situations. What would be said of a pianist who
could only perform *cadenza* passages of a particular type?
If only dancing were considered as an expressive art, and
not as an exhibition of acrobatic effects, if only it were
judged on the same plane as the other arts, how
soon would the poverty of its resources and the mental,
moral, and artistic inferiority of some of its exponents be
apparent!

In every art there exist several techniques that are but
rarely associated in one individual. May not one prefer
that which gives naturalness of expression, simplicity of
demeanour and harmony of vital functions? Such a technique is not directed to external effects, but by means of it
the artist can bring into entire agreement his faculties
of impulsion, reflection and harmonious creation.

At the beginning of the present century, gymnastics
consisted entirely of staccato movements of the body,
arrested in their motor impulses and effected at traditional
speeds. The points of departure and arrival were con-
fused; the qualities of elasticity were very little sought;
straight or angular movements succeeded one another
abruptly, without preparation or connection, while curved
lines were neglected or ignored. Each limb was to be
exercised in a certain number of determined positions and
each category of exercises was complete in itself. The
influence of this gymnastic training with its angularity of
outline and its short and sharply-defined metres made itself
felt in dramatic art, above all in the lyric theatre. The
actors did not follow the melodic line in their movements;
they were content by means of gestures or pauses to
emphasise the beginnings and endings of the musical

phrases; and in Wagnerian opera, for example, the gestures designed by the composer (as in the forging scene in Siegfried, etc.) often appeared to arrive too late, because they were only perceived by the spectator at the actual moment when they were due, the singers not having cultivated the art of preparing them mentally.

All gesture is the result either of an immediate exaltation or of a persistent state of emotion, or, again, of a conscious thought voluntarily pursued. In some cases the sensory organs use all their powers of elastic expansion to project the thought outwards. In other cases the mind tries to eliminate sensation in order better to concentrate itself, thus involving a drawing-in or compression of the body before the logically expected impulse. Again, idea and sensation may be united by a series of calm waves which create psycho-physical balance.

Thus there exist gestures of expansion, of situation, of explanation and of decoration, gestures immediately accentuating tonic accents, as also those of slow pursuit of a train of thought. These gestures rise spontaneously from the depths of our being, of which they externalise the motor impulses and the sudden changes of intention, or manifest the slow evolution of an emotion by means of a series of nuances (*i.e.* little rhythms of hand, arm, shoulder, head, connected with the more complete rhythms involving displacements of the body), which create the big rhythms of the whole individual, and unite the straight, curved and broken lines of the human body. Bonds of connection ought to exist between the movements of the body, "bridges" between their point of origin and their point of arrival, if they are to have an æsthetic value and to convey emotion and sentiment with suppleness and elasticity. In other words, periods of continuity and solidarity must be created in gesture.

F

It was in this way that in 1905, struck by the stiffness of the usual gymnastic movements, I conceived *continuous bodily movements*, analogous to those of the bow on the

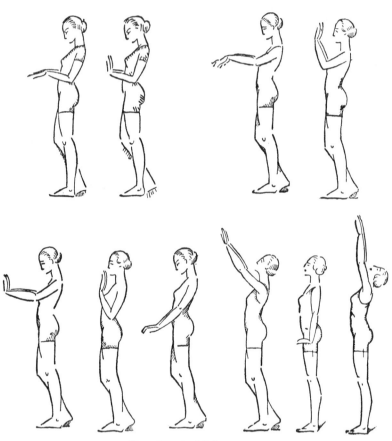

FIG. 20. – Slow Vertical Movements of Arms

string, or a sustained sound on a wind instrument. The slowness of these continuous movements is the product of muscular resistance. I caused them first to be practised separately and then connected them with arrested movements in order, finally, to have them executed in conjunction with these latter (polyrhythm). This new technique has gradually supplanted the old, and the reform of

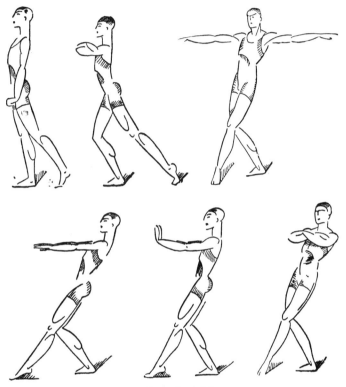

FIG. 21. – Slow Leg Movements

gymnastic teaching is now completed by exercises purely musical in essence, suggested by "rhythmic gymnastics."

This must be affirmed once for all, since so many teachers make a point of ignoring our efforts.

If the pianist's *legato* is studied under the microscope, as it were, it is found that each sound is connected to the following one by a continuous movement of the fingers,

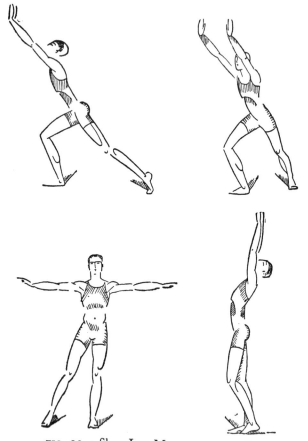

FIG. 22. – Slow Leg Movements – *contd.*

hand and wrist. These same fingers can effect slow curves in writing or drawing. The longer limbs can move so slowly that their displacement seems imperceptible. Even the facial muscles can contract and relax in uninterrupted movement (their working may be perceived in a cinema "close-up," when the actor exhibits the gamut of his expressive changes of physiognomy). But the sensations evoked by continuous movements such as these are comparatively slight and do not affect the whole body, whereas those engendered by movements of the heavier parts of the body – arms, legs and trunk – work through the whole organism and constitute a kind of internal "massage" of the individual. Any rhythm resulting from alternate muscular contraction and expansion will awaken another rhythm in the neighbouring muscular groups, and these again others in all parts of one's being. It is therefore indispensable that the teaching of gymnastics should include, in addition to the traditional exercises, a series of studies of the currents uniting the points of departure and arrival of bodily movements, in all degrees of speed and energy. The individual is thus aware of three sensations: that of setting the gesture in motion, that of the course of the gesture and that of its termination, whereas in classical gymnastics the only sensations experienced are those of the beginning and end of the movements. The character of these sensations is entirely changed according to which part of the limb moved is first put into action, and, again, according to the choice of the limb which originates a general movement. Thus, a movement of the arm may originate in the upper arm, elbow, hand, or finger. The arm, being attached to the trunk, may entail a movement of this also, while in other cases a movement of the trunk may be brought about by a turning movement of the hips or legs. The trunk can, in its turn, cause the arms to move, on account of their connection with it by means of the scapular and clavicular system, etc.

The study of continuous movements is closely connected with that of the elastic possibilities of the limbs, which vary in suppleness and energy according to the duration of the movements to be effected, and also according to the force of the motor impulse which brings about the movement. This impulse can be reduced to such a minimum of energy as entirely to escape analysis, or, on the other hand, it may be so vigorous that all parts of the body are irresistibly stimulated to movement in various rhythms, simultaneous or successive. Consequently, the study of motor impulses forms a very important element in physical education. Since 1905, I have caused them to be executed, under the name of "motor anacruses," and I have tried to determine their influence on gestures and attitudes according to the variation of their duration, energy and relation with space, and the degrees of all three rhythmic factors combined (*viz.* agogism, dynamism, and spatial dimension).

It is curious to note the difference that exists between the essential principles of the present stage of musical evolution and those of present-day physical education. In the domain of living plastic the young man of to-day endeavours to escape from anything of an intellectual nature. Physical education seeks to excite a general impulse of the body, the origin of the motor faculties, spontaneous gesture born of muscular imagination, passion and fantasy. In music, on the contrary, the present generation is in revolt against sentiment and emotion. Its researches seem to be inspired purely by considerations of order and æsthetics. Education is consequently obliged to combat this Apollonian state of mind and to arouse the qualities of emotion and sensibility in the musical apprentice. It is by a series of continuous movements performed, so to speak, in the depths of consciousness that the inner impulses gradually come to the surface and are capable of being externalised in an æsthetic and orderly fashion.

The question of *tempo* plays an important part in the

technique of continuous movement. At a very rapid pace the successive impulses finally lose their force; at too slow a speed they break up the movement. It is therefore

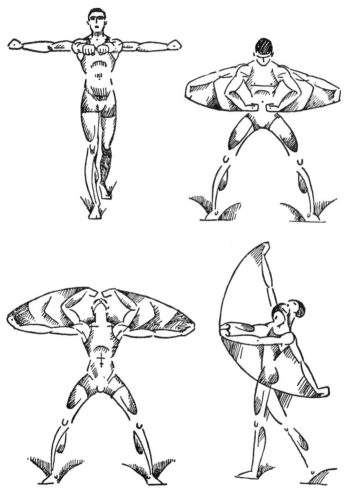

FIG. 23. – Exercises in Slow Shifting of the Weight of the Body (on the Spot)

necessary carefully to measure the degrees of moderate *tempo* in such a way as to make the influence of the first impulse last, and also to ensure the continuity of the movement by means of secondary impulses of a similar nature. Breathing, judiciously but not artificially regulated, ensures the character of the motor impulses and their natural connection. There is a great difference between a number of rhythmic fragments connected by

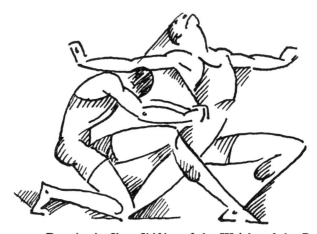

FIG. 24. – Exercise in Slow Shifting of the Weight of the Body
(on the Spot)

a continuous movement and a sustained and uninterrupted rhythm imperceptibly phrased by successive impulses. Simple impulses are not sufficient to create a physical style, and the error of certain present-day systems of physical culture seems to me to lie in merely giving different forms to the impulses of the individual without either studying their consequences or placing them in the plastic phrase from the point of view of anacrusis. It ought not to be possible to separate a motor impulse from its metacrusis.

Once the nature of the anacrusic impulses and of the movements which result therefrom is determined, there remains the study of how to terminate the movement, to place the limb executing it in a certain plane or degree of space, then to regulate the dynamic degrees of muscular contraction at the moment of halting. The movement may either be definitely terminated or allowed gradually to exhaust itself after a crescendo or decrescendo of

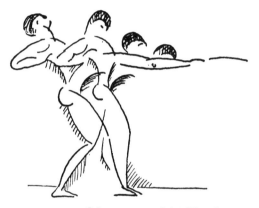

FIG. 25. – Movements of the Trunk

energy; it may be connected with a new impulse which will cause it to rebound in another direction or return to the first; it may be definitely arrested at the end of its trajectory or interrupted in mid-course, before the limb has traversed all the space open to it. When the nature of impulses and arrests has been sufficiently analysed to allow the points of departure and arrival of movements to harmonise quite naturally, then must be studied the form of the connecting lines between ictus and terminus. These lines, which may be straight, curved or broken, will be traced in all the space surrounding the body in static position. Exercises in slow bending, stretching and turning will increase the range of straight or rounded lines, spiral movements ensuring the possibility of continuation to infinity. And lines may be traced in space by the arms and the trunk while walking or running, whose course may either follow or direct that of the moving feet, and "melodies" as simple and varied as those created by a succession of musical sounds may be traced in space by the evolutions of the body.

It is difficult to realise the extraordinary variety of research relative to the creation of scales of continuous movement, and of ways of associating them. When this study is sufficiently advanced it must be completed by that

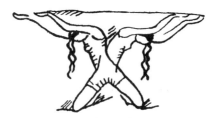

FIG. 26. – Slow Circumduction of Trunk

of the relations between continuous movements and those arrested and fixed, whether executed synchronously by different limbs, or whether *legato*, continuous gestures are combined with a counterpoint of *staccato* gestures and *vice versa*. A vast number of possible combinations suggest themselves: change of point of arrival during the course of the gesture; change of choice of leading muscular group; change of *tempo* (one arm twice or three times as fast, for example); change of amplitude of gesture (one arm describing the same figure as the other but reduced in scope by half or a quarter); etc., etc. The lines may be traced with special objects, such as sticks, batons, stretched cords, balls or balloons rolled on the

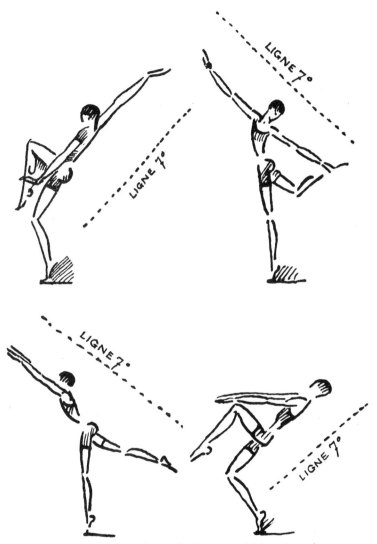

FIG. 27. - Running with Changes of Line (p. 74)

floor; they may be done on stairs or inclined planes, during leaps or in recumbent position. . . . If a single individual has so many different motor resources at his disposal, what may not be possible when his gestures are allied to those of one or two partners or a group? In this connection the combinations of musical polyphony, polyrhythm and polymetre give us invaluable indications for gestures and evolutions of human groups. Canons of lines, files, circles, opposing movements of lines and files,

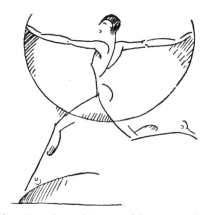

FIG. 28. – Running with Arm Movements (p. 74)

geometrical or pictorial designs, association or dissociation of bending and rising, contrasts of continuous movements on the spot and of interrupted running movements, leaps, crouching, etc. All this constitutes a veritable living symphony, a dynamic and spatial art impregnated with moving life. A great field of activity is henceforth open to dramatic and choreographic artists, and already the *mise en scène* of the Russian ballets betrays interesting researches (*e.g. Pas d'Acier*, Prokofieff) in the domain of polyrhythm.

On the other hand, the classical ballet, although sometimes influenced *externally* by the experiments being tried at present, wears threadbare its continual effects of jerky

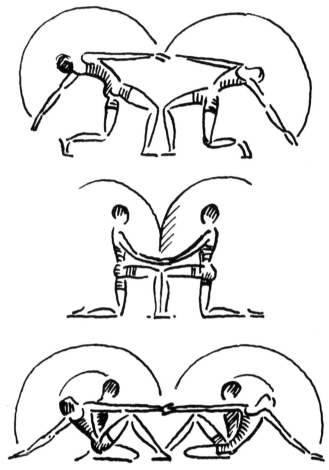

FIG. 29. – Series of Slow Movements by Two Partners

movements, leaps and voltes. It is very rare to find a dancer capable of continuous movements. Furthermore, the stereotyped movements of the traditional ballet are executed within an incredibly small range of *tempi*. They

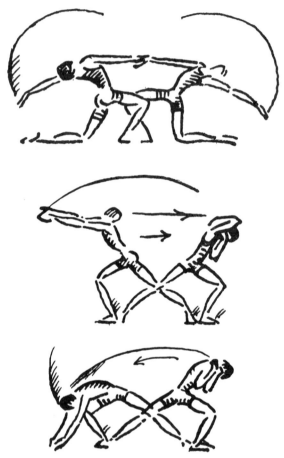

FIG. 30. – Series of Slow Movements by Two Partners – *contd.*

are certainly performed in exact time, since they are accompanied by orchestra, but they have become so automatic that they can only be executed at a fixed rate of speed. Effects of *accelerando* and *ritardando*, *crescendo* and *decrescendo* are very difficult to obtain in ballet to-day, because dancers only study gestures and leaps for their own sake, without the smallest desire to put this admirable technique at the service of a continuous idea. Continuous toe-walking is evidently an attempt at continuous movement, but this toe-work is so unnatural that it can never give that impression of sustained calm which lies in the serene and tranquil succession of connected slow movements.

In short, the error of present-day classical dancers lies in their being unable, and even unwilling, to adapt their technique to the artistic mentality of our age. The excellence of the choreographic physical exercises cannot be denied, but the art of to-day demands a more complete independence of movement, a greater suppleness in the connection of rhythms, a more alertly sensitive musicality and a more elastic accommodation to changes of *tempo* than formerly.

The movements of traditional dancing are little varied, and are no longer of interest to-day, except when employed and transfigured by a strong artistic personality. Happily there exist certain classical dancers who endeavour to transform their technique to enable it to meet new æsthetic requirements, but the classical school as a whole remains entirely stationary, and dance-students have to be content with a restricted education reduced to the practice of old-fashioned choreographic and rhythmic exercises, which make no attempt either to develop their artistic instinct and temperament or to arouse their imagination or form their character and personality.

In the theatre, especially in the cinema theatre, many actors have an intuitive sense of continuous movement, but attempts at harmonising a group of persons are rarely

made, nor are they possible until each individual actor
has studied the laws of continuous movement. Consider

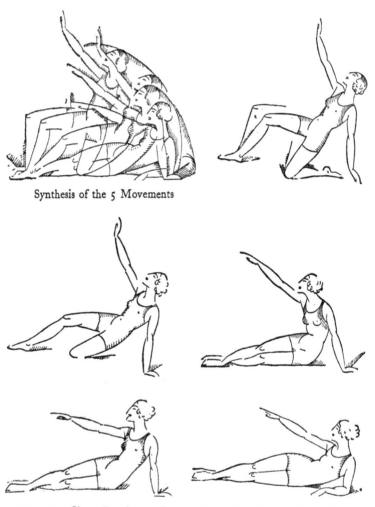

Synthesis of the 5 Movements

FIG. 31. – Slow Continuous Passage from Kneeling to Recumbent
Position

simple changes of stage position. The actor has to move from one point and take up a position at another. This is a continuous movement, created by his *inner* impulse, which connects the starting-point of his steps with their termination. This impulse is the result either of an emotion or of a state of reflection and analysis, and is continued by the will, which sustains the steps in a style suited to the dramatic action (such as ecstasy, passion, revolt, timid desire, etc.), the style being created by voluntary modifications of the usual gait. Sometimes the continuity of the steps is interrupted by a "resistance," and a new impulse is required to recommence. Resistance creates a reaction. A continuous movement may be composed of a whole series of little movements connected by a leading idea. If the pause is prolonged the body must remain in a state of balance, and antagonistic muscular forces must be harmoniously regulated according to the length of the pause. The vitality of group evolutions is born of the contrasts created by the different types of gait and deportment of the individual performers. In comparison with the thorough study of physical technique considered necessary for instrumentalists and conductors, this study in dramatic training is neglected to an astonishing extent.

To live life fully both mind and body must be free. Physical and intellectual liberty are not exclusively evidenced in expansive fashion by primitive impulses; the steady pursuit of an idea, as also the slow, elastic and measured development of a movement, give evidence of the free possession of a clairvoyant, prevoyant mind, which knows how to skirt obstacles and choose out new paths, always with a clear perception of the goal to be reached.

A sustained rhythm demands great suppleness of execution, an elastic promptitude, in cases where rapid

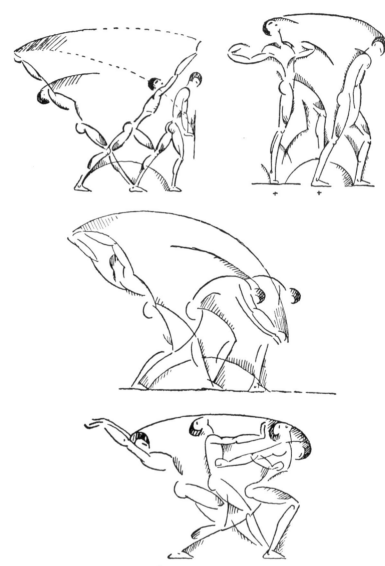

FIG. 32. – Successions of Movements

and unexpected changes of direction arise. To quit one point in order to reach another, choosing, in doing so, the best path, is, in short, to act rhythmically. Untimely stops created by reflection, anxiety or fatigue introduce into the rhythmic current resistances which change its form, and are capable of creating picturesque effects, but these should not compromise the sure progression to the end pursued, and both the mind, on the one hand, and the nervous and muscular systems on the other, should be ready to create connections between the subsidiary currents and to assure the arrival of the principal current at its goal.

It is important that the educator should endeavour to develop the temperament and character of his pupils as they are revealed in the four periods of childhood and adolescence, to restore wholly to the body the primitive rhythms of the personality, to combat all resistances, intellectual and physical, to correct their faults or turn them into good qualities. Too often, on the contrary, he only modifies the appearance of the character and develops the secondary rhythms, instead of searching into the depths of their being for the source of a principal rhythmic current by means of which the whole of their faculties may be uniformly developed.

Unfortunately, the aim of education is often considered to be the developing of children to maturity in the shortest possible time: education hastens to make them into men. This is a noble aim, and undoubtedly the educator's task is largely to depart from the present in order to prepare and assure the future, but is it not of primary importance to assure the present and to allow the child to develop all the qualities of his age, to procure for him the innocent joys which should keep alive his freshness and his curiosity? If these joys are complete their memory will cast a fragrance over his whole life. And it is equally necessary

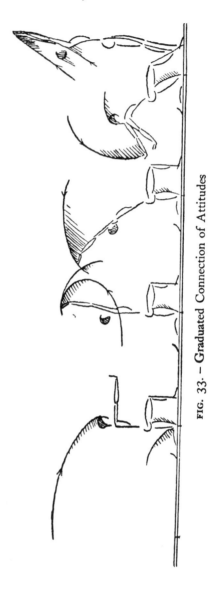

FIG. 33. – Graduated Connection of Attitudes

to enable young people at the period of adolescence to live their lives wholly and freely before demanding of them constant sacrifices to reason and tradition. Qualities of maturity are frequently required of them which time alone can develop. In trying to make them logical we run the risk of drying up the sources of their enthusiasm, smothering their innate need of ideals. . . .

Continuous movements are not natural to the earliest years. The child's natural form of expression is

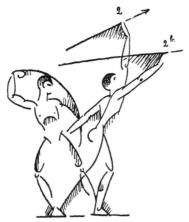

FIG. 34. – Connection of Movements Facing and in Profile

spasmodic, with no solid links between gesture and idea. He proceeds by leaps and jumps; he does not prepare future actions, he often forgets present ones. This constant *staccato* is not a fault: it betrays a natural state of elasticity and rebound; and to seek to develop unduly in him the sensation of and feeling for continuous movement would be as erroneous as to make him read Bergson, or listen to the later Beethoven sonatas. The negro – a grown-up child – instinctively avoids continuous movements. Vivid and characteristic as are his nervous, jerky

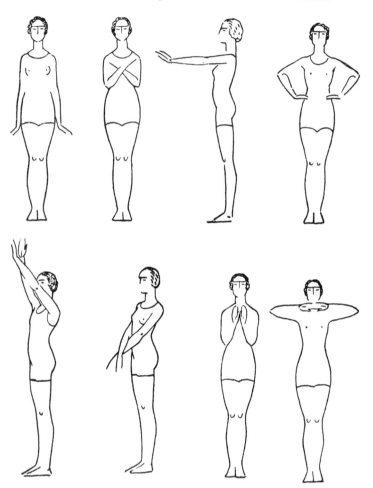

FIG. 35. – Slow Articulation of Limbs

dances, would not the slow and rounded gestures of
Isadora Duncan look ridiculous in him?

The child, both in play and in reasoning, lacks a sense
of continuity and development. His attention is solicited

at every instant by so many interesting curiosities, he
experiences so many sensations continually renewed, that
he has no time to make choice between all these riches,
and contents himself with enjoying them successively,

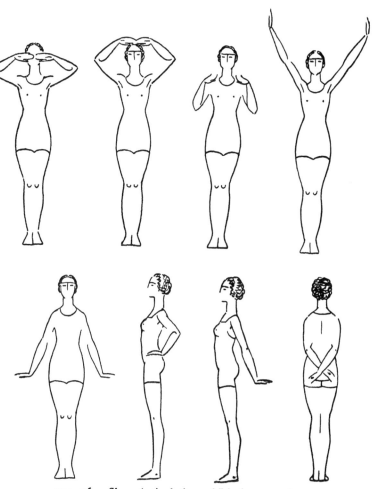

FIG. 36. – Slow Articulation of Limbs – *contd.*

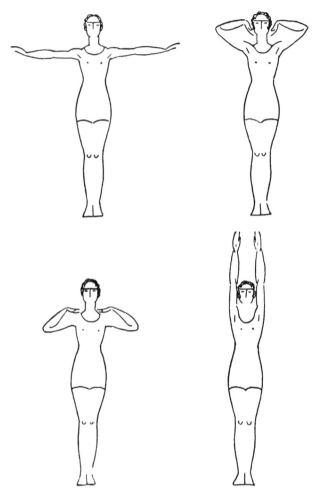

FIG. 37. – Slow Articulation of Limbs – *contd.*

never stopping to reflect. Early childhood is the age of improvisation, *i.e.* of spontaneous creation. The task of the educator is to ensure to the child the possession of the greatest possible number of full sensations. In the special domain of physio-rhythmic education, the child should be introduced more particularly to decided, prompt, short and rapid movements, and should be continually incited to discover for himself his most significant motor powers. He should be taught to make rapid connections between certain movements, to order them exactly and grade them according to his fancy. His spontaneous impulses should be cultivated and increased in number, those that are harmful or useless being eliminated. He should be taught

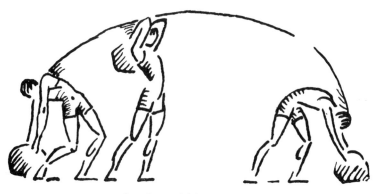

FIG. 38. – Lateral Transfer of Weight

principally the straight path from one point to another, avoiding too frequent movement in broken lines. To get the feeling of the great elementary rhythms, it is important to avoid encumbering the big definite lines with a multitude of small contradictory ones. Too often in traditional education the child's brain is crammed with such a quantity that his mind has difficulty in tracing a direction. The brain does not possess sufficient power of *dilatation* to prevent encumbrances being produced in it! Fragments of knowledge get entangled, directions are hindered. In the departure of a movement there is no certainty of preparation or unity in launching it, new acquisitions do not complete previous ones, they sometimes even annihilate them. The problems given to children should be quite simple, and should be chosen in such a way that the attacking of one may at the same time develop the capacity to solve others. The uncertainty created in physical domains by broken lines will cause the intellect to suffer correspondingly. Nothing further than assuring the impulse generating a movement

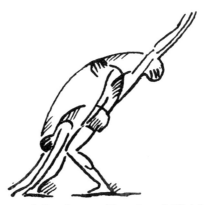

FIG. 39. – Slow and Continuous Transfer of Weight Backwards

should be required of children. It is bad teaching continually to demand the mental effort necessary to prepare consciously a bodily rhythm, to regulate its course slowly, and to make it terminate in special conditions of energy or duration. If such an effort is occasionally required of the child, it should be reduced to a minimum, and the aim should be well within his reach.

For the adolescent, exercises in slow and continuous movement will be very salutary from all points of view, for they demand concentration of mind, physical and moral balance and will-power. They develop instinct at

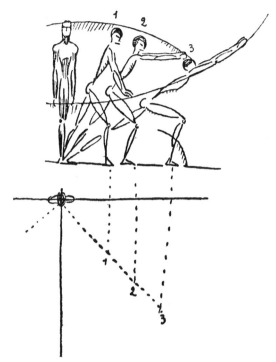

FIG. 40. – Examples of Lunges

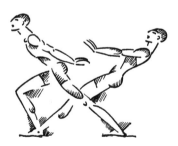

FIG. 41. – Lunges Forward and Backward with partial Transfer
of Weight of the Body

the same time as reflection, and assure the harmony of the vital functions. Youth lives intensely, ignorant of its tendencies and of its faults, its powers and imperfections. The adolescent must be enabled to regulate freely his muscular antagonisms and the play of his nervous currents,

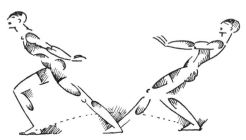

FIG. 42. – Backward and Forward Lunges with Transfer of the Whole Weight and a large Step

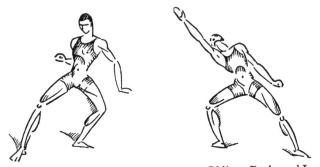

FIG. 43. – Lunge to the Side   FIG. 44. – Oblique Backward Lunge

to reduce his efforts to a strict minimum and economise his impulses, to measure instinctively the distance between the point in space where his gesture is prepared and the goal which it is proposing to reach. He must calmly survey the developments of the big initial rhythm and of the smaller secondary rhythms connected with it. Thus does he promote the harmonisation of his faculties; his mind is impregnated with a feeling of perfect balance, born of the peaceful sensation created by the balance of the physical forces. Each of his faculties is thus given the task for which it is fitted, in order that, as biologists tell us, instincts shall not be substituted for feelings, nor these for intelligence, nor this, again, for feelings or instincts. . . .

This general harmony of our cerebral, physical and spiritual forces assures for us the free possession of ourselves, develops our imagination, and quite naturally transports our sensations and feelings, conceptions and actions, into the domain of art. Art is in intimate correlation with life: it is the outward projection of love and the knowledge of beauty and truth.

EDUCATION

V

GENERAL EDUCATION AND RHYTHMIC MOVEMENT

EDUCATION does not consist in creating faculties which the pupil does not possess, but rather in enabling him to obtain the utmost possible benefit from those he does possess. The teacher who succeeds in this difficult task will at the same time develop freedom of action and thought in his pupils, thus stimulating them in the direction of creative effort. To attain this end, all teachers should understand the difference between instruction and education. Instruction is passive; it is a means of accumulating knowledge. Education is an active force working upon the will and tending to co-ordinate the various vital functions. The teaching profession has fallen into disfavour on the Continent more than in England. It is nevertheless well to remember that many of the finest intellects have grappled with the problems of child-education. We recall Plato, Fénelon, Montaigne, Rousseau, Spencer, Goethe, and Schiller, to mention only a few, and the remarkable thing is that all agree in regarding early childhood as the critical – and so the most interesting – period from the educational standpoint.

One of the most recent developments in educational theory regards education as the study of physical and moral qualities in their relation to life. It is not so long ago that the child was found to have a sort of physical consciousness, one that had been too long and too utterly neglected. In certain recent textbooks, indeed, I have come across the expression "rhythmic education," but on closer examination I have found the words corresponded to no practical reality whatsoever. My practical experience is that the majority of the children I teach have not been prepared for the kind of instruction I wish to give them. Of course one does not expect to find the body of a child of five or six years of age perfectly formed and fully developed; but one is frequently amazed to note how greatly it has been neglected during the first few years of life.

From about the age of ten months the child learns to imitate the movements shown him and also to link on some idea to each movement. The utmost possible advantage should be taken of this natural aptitude. A baby, for instance, cannot too soon begin to understand the meaning of "right" or "left." In teaching him it is not enough to point to his right hand and then to one's own, while saying "right." At a very early age the child should be taught the meaning of direction by his teacher standing behind him and making him bend the whole of his body to right and to left. Every movement should be encouraged; yet parents frequently make the mistake of completely neglecting this phase of education. Children ought to be urged and encouraged to move, not only their arms in response to a word or an idea, but also their legs, head, neck, shoulders, eyes, etc. They should learn the meaning of "horizontal" and of "vertical" by being made to lie flat on the ground and then to stand upright. The parents' words should rouse their motor consciousness; simultaneously with the growth of this particular consciousness will develop the power to perform each of the movements dwelt on in mind. It often happens that parents attach too much importance to certain special organs, with the result that other organs are neglected. For instance, they educate a child's ear and neglect his eye. Very few children are trained to distinguish the various shades of one and the same colour. As regards the ear, it is of utmost importance, in my opinion, to teach children to distinguish, not only the various steps of the musical scale, but also the direction from which a sound comes: in front or from behind, above or below. What distance has the sound traversed? What is its intensity? A child is enormously interested in any game which appeals to his instinct for analysis. It is important then to utilise this tendency, and to keep his curiosity constantly alert by supplying him with fresh subjects for analysis – in the form of amusement, of course, and taking every precaution against brain fatigue.

To return to the problem of movements of the body. It is a matter of regret that so few mothers know anything about anatomy. Occasionally indeed it happens that even specialists are incredibly ignorant on this matter. By "specialists" I mean, for instance, teachers of the piano who know absolutely nothing of the mechanism of the hand, or masters of singing who know the larynx only by name. A mother who is instructed in the anatomy of her child's body will assuredly stimulate quite instinctively a far greater variety of movements in the child than will a more ignorant mother. One can never insist too much on the importance of unreservedly encouraging children, from earliest infancy, to experiment in all their powers of contraction and relaxation, of motion at varying degrees of speed, etc. The greater and more diversified the child's physical experience, the more numerous the facets, so to speak, which will reflect his imagination. The sure result – in addition to an excellent physical development – will be a certain intellectual quickening that consists of the faculty of benefiting by experience. No sooner has the child experimented on a number of movements than he unconsciously begins to classify them and to choose those most useful to him. The power of choice is the basis of the sense of freedom. If a child knows only one way to do some particular thing, his action is compulsory in its nature; he ceases to be a free agent. As an instance of early educational routine – all babies, at birth, are potentially ambidextrous; yet, taking children of seven years of age, scarcely more than one per cent will be found to have developed this potentiality. One need not insist on the advantage of displaying the same skill in both limbs symmetrically, instead of imposing on a single hand the task of working for both. It is also unnecessary to dwell on the fact that the parallel development of both hands naturally implies superior equilibrium.

In the instruction of quite small children, what I call inhibition exercises should not be neglected. All the same, I would recommend parents not to check a movement of their children except for a definite purpose: for example, to attract their attention or to make them imitate a fresh movement. The development of attention in children tends to strengthen their brain-capacity. It is as important for the child to be able to fix his attention instantaneously as it is to avoid strain upon it. Thirty seconds of attention at a time is sufficient for a child of twelve months; from two to three minutes should be regarded as a maximum for a child between two and three years of age. The natural qualities which benefit by education of the attention are chiefly memory and concentration; and the best means of training the attention of children is to play intelligently with them. Games should be joy-giving; I look upon joy as the most powerful of all mental stimuli.

It is, therefore, erroneous to imagine that the task of parents has come to an end when the child begins to play. On the other hand, no action retains its virtue as a stimulus if repeated so frequently as to become automatic.

This is why care should be taken to have the greatest possible variety of games played, and why every opportunity should be seized of introducing fresh elements. Lack of variety brings about stagnation. The ideal form of play is that between two children: the second child supplies opportunities for emulation. The main thing to remember is that the function of parents and teachers is to strengthen and develop the child in such fashion that mind and body form a perfect instrument whereon to learn to play the song of life.

The period of child-development dealt with up to this point is the one preceding the time when the child becomes really capable of thinking. When this moment arrives, he begins to observe his sensations and gradually learns to co-ordinate them. If at the same time he has the chance of being taught rhythmic movement, he learns not only to set up relations between his acts, but to give them an object definitely perceived, thus strengthening his will-power. The greater the variety of movements taught him by his mother, the better equipped will he be for taking full advantage of the lessons both of school and of life itself. And when this truth has become more widely known and practised, there will come about a considerable amelioration in the human race, and the many problems of education will be more easy to solve. For, after all, the aim of education is to do away with harmful and useless habits, to encourage those that are beneficial and profitable. Brain, nerves, and muscles ought to thrill with an intense vital stream, whose function it is to transmit sensations, emotions, and ideas. The power that sends forth this stream and regulates its output is rhythm — sovereign master of movement and rest, of sound and silence, light and shade, joy and pain, defeat and victory.

Charles Lalo says, somewhere, that rhythm is a muscular phenomenon. To this I would add that the rhythmic instinct is the ability, which our muscular system possesses, of perceiving the duration and the gradations of bodily movements, and that the science of rhythm is the power of appreciating the relations of movements to one another, of bringing measured movements under the control of the mind. Rhythm, consequently, is by no means an exclusive apanage of the musical art. Indeed, the teaching of rhythmic movement, although based on music, is not solely a preparation for musical studies, but rather a system of general culture. The Greeks attached great importance to rhythmic movements: they recognised the beneficent influence of a rhythmic education of both body and mind, and they also knew that this rhythmic education was capable of influencing the inner life of man. Plato says:

"Rhythm, *i.e.* the expression of order and symmetry, penetrates by way of the body into the soul and into the entire man, revealing to him the harmony of his whole personality."

Clearly, the musician will greatly benefit from studies in rhythmic movement, though these will be equally beneficial to the future painter or to any other future creator. Musicians who are anxious to teach it will possess at the outset only one superiority over other classes of artists from the rhythmic point of view: they will already be familiar with time-notation and with certain other intellectual elements. But, on the whole, the simple knowledge of music does not constitute a preparation more favourable to the study of rhythmic movement than does the simple knowledge of bodily rhythms to the study of rhythmic sounds. Rhythm and sound ought to complement each other, just as in the study of the fine arts, rhythm, line and colour complement each other. The aim of rhythmic gymnastics is to develop mind and feeling in everything connected with art and life. Its study is all the more indispensable to the musician since music without rhythm is lifeless, whereas rhythm and movement are essential factors of every form of art, and are indispensable to every thoroughly cultured human being. Consequently, the study of the laws of motion is necessary for every child, as well as for teachers and parents.

Children are of widely differing temperaments, and the relations between the movements of each particular child differ accordingly. Some children are restless, others apathetic; some always strained, others limp and flaccid.* Some, unbalanced in gait, will be found to be unbalanced in reasoning power; others, incapable of stepping to music without lagging at each step, will be found to have difficulty in following a discussion or an explanation; others, again, who hurry ahead as they advance, pass their emotional and intellectual life in precipitate excitement. These differences of character should be observed and taken into consideration; for if children do not learn to struggle against the defects of their nature, they will commit faults which will hinder and retard their development throughout life.

It is sad to note how few completely normal children there are in a class. What different forms may be assumed by that malady — so serious and yet so seldom analysed and treated by doctors — which has been given the name of *arhythm*. This is due to disharmony between the cerebral driving machinery and the practical motor forces. At the outset of my experiments I was content to bring regularity into gait and gesture, to force the body to act accordingly. Then, discovering that the irregularity was often the resultant of insufficient spontaneity in motor rhythm, I instituted alternating experiences, some of which aim at arousing and exciting the temperament,

* See "The Inner Technique of Rhythm," p. 52.

developing the muscular elasticity without which no nervous reaction can impart a complete impulse to the motor system – while the rest, once the impulsive faculties are unconsciously and unreasoningly developed, aim at harmonising and co-ordinating them in accordance with the laws that control the relations between time, space, and dynamic force.

It is important that exercises for children should not be chosen in haphazard fashion. In my system, each lesson is most carefully broken up into distinct "chapters," as it were, and to teach it properly each chapter should figure in every lesson, even though it be as a single exercise. This latter, however, should always be given to the child in the two ways described above, *i.e.* first, to awaken spontaneity of mind and body, and diminish the interval of time between the conception of an act and its realisation; second, to bring order into the child's spontaneous bodily manifestations. I have had occasion to give lessons to a large number of ultra-nervous children, suffering from too frequent contractions and irregular decontractions or from too deep-rooted vital expansions (*i.e.* from too rapid and complete exhaustion), and others incapable of rapid impulsions, or of natural successions of quick and slow movements. The constant tendency of the intellectual centres to control the motor apparatus produces a state of irritation, discouragement, and lack of self-confidence which only increases the nervous disturbance. All this results in obsessions which interrupt normal life and end in creating imaginary diseases.

It was my teachers' classes that showed me the manifest power of rhythmic gymnastics in transforming the mind along the lines of greater self-possession, stronger power of imagination, more constant mental concentration. Did this mean that children could not profit, equally with adults, from eurhythmics? By no means: but the effect of my exercises was inevitably feebler when lessons were few and far between (two lessons per week are insufficient to cure abnormal children) than in classes where eurhythmics is practised for two hours each day. Consequently, in future I shall carry on my work by attempting to introduce rhythmic gymnastics into the elementary schools, with one daily lesson of fifteen or twenty minutes, or perhaps four half-hour lessons per week.* Under these conditions, I imagine that motor habits will become regularly established in five or six years. Naturally, such an upheaval of the school syllabus will not come about without a severe struggle. It seems to me, however, that if nerve specialists would be good enough to study my experiments carefully, they would speedily recognise the therapeutic value of exercises that control muscular contraction and relaxation, in every shade of time, energy and space, for instruction thus given must inevitably stimulate intuition and endow the pupils with bodies perfectly organised, both mentally and physically.

It is unnecessary to remind educationists how wide is their field of action if they aim at performing their task in a manner creditable to their profession; but I should like to recommend to their notice one of the criteria I apply to myself. I ask myself: "Am I content, I whose task it is to educate tiny children and prepare them for the future?" Confronted with this question, we are all sometimes constrained to bow the head in silence. On the other hand, when we are able to leave the class with the feeling that we have given of our best, and have done all we could to put before the coming generation an ideal towards which we, for the most part, have but vainly tried to reach, then we can exclaim with conviction and in all earnestness: "Yes, I am content, perfectly content."

* The results obtained in certain village schools of Switzerland are perfectly satisfactory.

VI

RHYTHM IN MUSICAL EDUCATION

NINE out of every ten children take up the study of a musical instrument without having music within themselves. Hence, the teacher has a dual task before him. He has to initiate into the mechanism of the instrument a muscular apparatus ignorant of its own mechanism, and also to bring his pupils into a condition to express, on an alien body, feelings which their own body has never experienced.

Before adapting his nature to the movement and sound of an instrument, the pupil should be capable of experiencing in his own body – and then of analysing – both motor and aural sensations; special exercises will first develop his sense of muscular rhythm and his nervous sensibility, then they will render his ear attentive to all gradations of intensity, duration and time, phrasing and shading, so that his limbs may faithfully reproduce the rhythms perceived by the ear. Hence the pupil will find himself in a better condition for motor receptivity, as well as better prepared to take up studies that aim at converting impression into expression. The teacher will then seek to diminish the time lost between impression and the faint desire for expression, by means of exercises whose object is to develop greater spontaneity both in the motor centres and in the imagination.* When all his movements have become rhythmical, a child learns to *think* and to express himself rhythmically. There can be

* See p. 110.

no distinct motor images in the brain unless the motor system is perfectly well organised.

Nor must it be forgotten that, from the musical point of view, the ear has two different tasks. The first is that of hearing rhythms separately and in association; the second is that of hearing sounds singly and in combination. The study of sound will begin when the ear becomes aware of the various gradations of rhythm and of time.* In both cases the series of exercises will be the same.

The voice will begin to imitate sound. Then the memory of sound movements will act on the mind and will call forth mental hearing. The ear listens to the external sound, the brain creates the inner sound, and so there comes into being the creative sense (improvisation, composition).

The pupil with a good ear is aware of the development of his powers of imagination. Mental hearing depends on sensation and memory, so that the art of sight-reading is based on a good receptive condition, on spontaneity of mind, and on certain powers of creative imagination, for mental hearing enables the pupil to build up intermediate sound-images that serve as bases for reading.

Once the child can hear, reproduce and read successions of rhythms and sounds, he will be initiated into musical *writing*. Then, possessed of the necessary qualities of receptivity and expression, *i.e.* ability to recognise sounds and movements, and to express rhythms and sounds in writing, he will be ready to take up the study of an instrument. His master will only have to teach him to transpose sounds and sound-images to strings or keyboard, by the aid of touch.

Twenty-five years ago, the study of solfège consisted exclusively in refining the faculty of sight-reading. The

* See "The Inner Technique of Rhythm," p. 51.

appearance of my method for developing the ear, the sense of hearing, and tonal feeling roused keen controversy in musical circles. The idea, however, has progressed, and excellent musicians, converted to these principles, have in turn invented interesting methods, whose aim is to fill up the *lacunæ* in the traditional teaching of solfège (formerly intended only for born musicians, mostly endowed with the faculty of absolute pitch) and to enable pupils with imperfect hearing to acquire *relative pitch.* . . . But this has not been so in the teaching of musical rhythm, and the various rhythmic systems that have appeared during the past ten years are, after all, no more than collections of processes aiming either at teaching metre to dancers or imparting to their movements a certain external grace.

One distinguishing characteristic of eurhythmics is that it evokes sensations which create mental images. Other educational methods differ from mine in confining themselves to the description of images, thus creating the illusion of sensations. I attempt to lay under contribution the physical body as a whole and so try to arouse in the muscular system a special sense of time by utilising the power to contract and relax the muscles. This power includes all degrees of strength, suppleness and rapidity. Rhythmic gymnastics starts from the principle that the body is the inseparable ally of the mind; it affirms that body and mind should harmoniously perform their divers functions, not only separately but simultaneously. The necessity for this simultaneity seems to derive from the dual nature of so many phenomena. Music, for instance, is not only the art of sound, but also that of accentuation and development in time; rhythm is not only the outcome of some intellectual process, it is a vital instinct. Our bodies are the vessels in which seethe our emotions, and our minds are the centres which inspire them with life. It is for the intellect to control the action of both. If we accept this analysis, we must also accept the existence, both in art and in life, of three forms of beauty which rhythm makes one: spiritual beauty, plastic beauty, and technical beauty. Combined, they appear as sensation, emotion and idea, expressed by the body, the heart and the brain.

Children are not taught to feel rhythm, but are merely told the signs that indicate it, the result being that the child becomes familiar with the effects of movement rather than with movement itself. Children learn to classify and name the various divisions of time; they acquire no personal experience of these divisions. The objection will be urged that any child who studies an instrument thereby becomes acquainted with that which eurhythmics is trying to teach him; but it can be proved that a purely digital acquaintance with rhythmic values is inadequate. Movement is not simply a matter of time, but also of accent and direction. Now, the sense of accent depends on a greater or less experience of muscular contractions, and direction depends on the starting-point of the various energies. If you leave it entirely to the fingers to create motor images in the mind, these images will inevitably remain feeble and incomplete. The whole body should come under the educational influence of rhythm, and it is greatly to be desired that this education should be given before the child has reached the age of nine, for after that age all that education can do will be to modify habits of mind and body that have already been acquired. The great difficulty which prevents the ideal of an education from being attained at the right time is found in the opposition of parents, and consequently in that of the heads of schools.

In practising our exercises, the pupils at once note an

appreciable delay between the motive will-power and its bodily interpretation. This is what Helmholtz has called "lost time." * The practice of rhythmic gymnastics tends to reduce this delay, and, by so doing, to strengthen volition, and to make the child more clearly aware of his power of bodily self-control. Gradually he will feel an increase in self-confidence, in his powers of execution, in those faculties which form a close and immediate link between will and act, between dream and life.

In his efforts to achieve rhythms by movement, the eurhythmist neophyte feels himself most powerfully aided by the music which accompanies the exercises. At first, he does not succeed in finding an exact equivalent for the different note-values in the rhythm of his movements. It would be a mistake to combat this sensation of inadequacy — except in the form of renewed energy and perseverance in the pursuit of a complete harmony. The discrepancy which the pupil observes between will and act possesses the advantage of making him aware of the hiatus between his mental and his physical habits. His problem therefore is as follows: how to set up agreement between mind and body? With a little practice he will be able to realise within himself movements in time and space; he will perceive the relation between the music of sounds and that of movement.

A striking phenomenon in lessons in eurhythmics is the extreme diversity of individual movements on the part of those who do the same exercises together, to the same music. In other words, there are great differences of interpretation of the same musical rhythms by different persons. This variety corresponds exactly to the personal characteristics of the various pupils, and it may be interesting to see why this individual factor, so striking in our classes, is absent in gymnastic or military exercises where

* See p. 106.

hundreds of individuals do the same movement in the same way. The reason is that the gestures of soldiers or gymnasts are an end in themselves, whereas those of our pupils are the manifestation of their higher will imposing certain rhythms on their bodily movements. Exercises in athletics or drill aim at a purely material object, whereas we endeavour to produce a common outward expression of individual emotions. Here rhythm is the link between mind and senses, and this to such a degree that each pupil speedily rejects the current opinion which looks upon the body as inferior to the mind. He quickly comes to regard his body as an instrument of incomparable delicacy, susceptible of the noblest and the most artistic expression.

Entire freedom should be given to the muscles of the foot and leg, as anyone who respects the laws of health will agree. Every pianist knows it would be impossible to acquire a good technique if one wore gloves while practising. The lack of anatomical knowledge of the human body, and of the habit of freely estimating its movements, as well as the constant anxiety of certain parents to prevent their children from seeing any object capable of reminding one of the academic human form – all this, instead of purifying the mind, disturbs and perverts it and makes it impure. Often have my pupils told me of the amazement of certain persons of their acquaintance on hearing that our rhythmic exercises take place with bare legs and feet! They found fault with this freedom of costume on the ground that it aroused evil thoughts. What answer can one give to such a reproach? Simply that pure-minded people do not harbour impure thoughts, and that if anyone is incited to evil thoughts by the sight of a naked leg, it is not the leg that must be blamed but rather his own mind, so ready to offer hospitality to unwholesome mental associations. Indeed, the sight and knowledge of the human form has never perturbed the mind of a child whose parents and teachers always regard it as innocent and natural.

The education of our several faculties continually brings us back to the same problem, whatever be the accomplishments or the failings of the individual. The painter should educate both hand and eye; the musician, both hand and ear, and so on. The general law is that each individual should learn to analyse and develop his ordinary talents and endeavour by exercise to overcome any opposition to the full development of his natural gifts.

Many are born with a sense of rhythm, though the power of expression is lacking: they have a well-organised brain which is ministered to by an inadequately educated or developed body. Those who, consciously or unconsciously, find themselves struggling with this conflicting force, are far more numerous than is generally imagined.

It is advisable to put teachers of children on their guard against a too widespread error: our system of education aims, not at repressing the unconscious movements which reveal the personality, but rather at making the muscular and nervous system so supple that these movements may express themselves in all their beauty. Rhythmic exercises are introduced only when the temperament is fully awakened, and the pupil is in complete control of his body. Indeed, it is useless to attempt to regulate imperfect movements, to examine inadequate sensations. Once the education of the nervous centres is finished, the pupil's natural rhythmic expression is impeded by no untimely conflicting force, his whole body is constantly ready to respond to sound rhythms. Then it is for the master to prevent this body from an excessive response, to introduce

moderation and orderliness into the subconscious rhythmic manifestations.

Once rhythm is awakened in body and brain, *i.e.* when
all sensation is ready to become thought and feeling, the
child is taught to blend his movements with those of
sound, to transpose the rhythms maintained by the whole
body into rhythms interpreted by the voice. He learns to
translate images of movement into images of sound,
which will be all the more distinct if the vocal action has
been more fully developed by technical exercises in
breathing, pitch and articulation. Finally, when the child
can write down what he has listened to and rhythmicised,
when he can read, *i.e.* bring sound before the mind,
guided solely by his mental hearing, the master will
introduce him to the instrument itself, teaching him to
apply to it the previously acquired faculties, through a
fresh transposition of sound-images.* The already
developed sense of rhythm becomes correlated with the
sense of touch. The general rhythmic technique becomes
specialised into a finger and arm technique. "Mental
rhythmical singing creates the external rhythmical
touch." † The child learns to imitate on the keyboard the
music singing within him, and so accustoms himself to a
new association of acts and thoughts: (1) to hear, to sing,
to play (imitation); (2) to think in sounds, to play (improvisation); (3) to read, to think in sounds, to play
(sight-reading).

It is clearly indispensable that the adapting of the
above-described preparatory studies to the instrument
should be made by the same professor or teacher, otherwise the unimaginative pupil runs the risk of not being
able, alone, to construct the bridge between the general

* See Chap. VII, "The Piano and Musicianship," p. 122.

† *La place de la méthode Jaques-Dalcroze dans les écoles populaires de
musique* (Nina Gorter).

I

and the specialised studies. The piano master who is not familiar with eurhythmics will not be able to utilise the resources possessed by his pupil. But if he is acquainted with the preparatory method, he is certain to advance the progress of the young eurhythmist at a very rapid pace, not only from the point of view of interpretation, but also in improvisation. He will have, in fact, to deal with a pupil who has already, from his own experience, learned that conscious analysis of muscular sensations, of spontaneous rhythms, and of realised sounds, gives full power of construction to the creative instinct.

Even were it to be disputed that eurhythmics gives pupils a clear and definite knowledge of musical rhythm and the power to practise it physically and instrumentally, I should still claim that it merits the consideration of all who have to teach children. Indeed, its practice gives to the child the physical sense of duration: the consciousness of the time required for contracting and relaxing his muscles. The pupil learns to know more than the sum total of his efforts; he learns to prove the relation that exists between each partial effort and all the rest. This knowledge enables him to gauge exactly the conflicting energy which prevents him from overcoming oppositions, and so to economise all superfluous expenditure of force. The exercises give the child perfect self-knowledge; they introduce order and harmony into his whole organism and dispel irrational nervous actions. He learns to see himself as he is objectively, is enabled to estimate his powers, is made aware of what he can accomplish. The result is a development of his imagination along healthy lines, and joy comes to him when he feels untrammelled by any physical inconvenience or mental preoccupation of a lower order. It is such joy to be able to act freely because he has rejected useless manifestations, to give himself up body and mind to the expression of feelings. He regains, so to speak, the virginity of vital elementary impressions. He is not ashamed to let himself go, because he knows that there has been created within him a regulating force which will keep him from excessive self-abandonment. And he joyfully gives himself up to the natural expansion of his feelings and sensations, because he feels that by fullness of life his whole nature becomes transformed. Thus, this joy is a new factor in moral progress, a new stimulant of the will.

This joy is evidently brought into being also by the fact that lessons are taken in common, to musical accompaniment. Music forges a link between the pupils. A multiple life animates every organism, constituting a single rhythm traversed by many currents, all differing in expansion, though inspired by one will. A sort of special atmosphere comes into being which fills each pupil with a quite individual sensation of solidarity. A force similar to that of electricity fills the room, linking the various organisms to one another. Frequently a single antagonistic thought or the fatigue of an individual breaks the charm and destroys the cohesion of all these agglomerated human rhythms, productive of one common rhythm that throbs with an intense collective life. The sense of being one in an ensemble of vibrant thoughts and wills momentarily destroys all personal preoccupation. Thus, in mixed classes, there takes place a kind of momentary desexualisation most favourable to the purification of individuals whose sense preoccupations encroach upon the desire for an harmonious, well-balanced life. In many cases, my pupils have been cured of *idées fixes*, of special obsessions, and many others have regained self-confidence once they learned to see clearly into their own body and mind, to grasp the relations that unite physical and intellectual rhythms.

In the first part of the lessons, musical and bodily rhythm are studied alone, without insistence on the relations between this dual rhythm and æsthetics. The pupils should simply seek after a precise bodily expression of the impressions they have received; then they observe and analyse the results. Though limiting the efforts of my pupils and myself to this preliminary task, I nevertheless insist on the fact that rhythm is a means, not an end in itself. Its function is to set up the relationship between the music we hear and that we have within ourselves. Our bodies are admirable instruments which are but waiting for us to allow them to react to the emotions they feel. Unfortunately, this reaction is almost always abortive at first in many pupils, and the emotion remains unexpressed for lack of the indispensable intermediary. This results in a suppression of forces ardently seeking expression and form. Absence of the power to express harmoniously emotions and impressions gives rise to a mental and bodily condition which is nothing less than chaotic. What is needed is simply rhythm, which is capable of expressing unconscious beauty, raising it to the level of art.

Psychologists have long since recognised how great an influence rhythmic movements are capable of exercising upon the brains of abnormal children. Naturally the influence is as great upon healthy children, possessed of a more complete power of relaxation. Muscular sensations enrich the brain, and man is at once both the possessor and the distributor of vital powers. To prevent himself from becoming the slave of these powers and to remain constantly their master, man has need of rhythm – the co-ordinating element of all his activities, that which creates a sympathetic current between his innumerable sensations and gives him a firm poise resulting from the balance it maintains between movement and rest.

Those who have come to understand the virtue of rhythm do not incur the risk of exhausting their emotions in vain efforts to express them bodily. It transposes these emotions on to a higher plane of being, where sensation is refined into feeling and the mind blends the elements of beauty into noble harmony, into an ideal instrumentation.

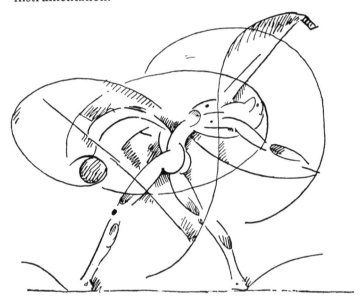

FIG. 45.—Movement of Arms and Trunk.

VII

THE PIANO AND MUSICIANSHIP
(1925)
(*To Mothers*)

Much has been written on the education of children in general, on musical education in particular. For a great mass of advice, infallible methods and systems, we are indebted to distinguished philosophers, professionals and professors, well-wishers of every kind. All have their own opinions as to the best way of teaching music to children. From time to time a congress or a public enquiry takes place, and musicians endeavour to agree on the matter. Then they return home, well pleased with themselves, and nothing further is heard of it.

Is there any way of sorting out this mass of opinion? We must first eliminate the opinions of those who have not been in frequent contact with children, and have not, with indefatigable interest and for a number of years, observed the natural development of their physical and moral powers. For only when we know the child can we tell what he will do. We have not even the right to give advice as to the education of a child of six if we have had dealings only with children of twelve. Systems of education ought to be modified according to the age of the children; the great defect of nine-tenths of the works on education is that they speak of children in the mass, without appearing to suspect that the child of five is a totally different individual from the boy or girl of ten, that at seven or eight years of age their individuality seems to have undergone a kind of reincarnation, and that therefore methods of instruction should follow the various phases of development. Theorists who have had no opportunity of analysing these different periods resemble an amateur naturalist making a series of observations on the skin of a serpent and the modifications introduced into its condition by age – continuing his observations throughout the life of the serpent, microscopically examining it every morning without noticing that it changes its skin every spring.

After eliminating all authors of works on musical education who have not acquired their information from personal experience, we have to do the same with theorists hidebound by tradition, chained to the past either by indolence or by business. Then there are the non-artists, those who consider only the externals of education, and teach only by rote or rule of thumb; and finally the utopists, those unable to prove, by producing children they have educated, that their method can be readily put into practice. It is a serious error to look upon life as so long that there is no need to make any sudden modification in our various conditions of existence. "We will see about it! . . ." "All things come to him who waits! . . ." "Let kindly Nature have her way! . . ." such are the expressions common both in family and in government routine. Unfortunately, their utterance irremediably compromises the future both of the children and of the adults of the present generations; for life will not wait, it follows its course, disdainful of human delay or hesitations, and the time comes when the child becomes a man, when the man will soon return to second childhood. Then we discover how much time we have squandered: we strive hard to recover it; but, alas, there is nothing to be done. We recognise that we have spent our time in quarrelling about words: that now it is too late to begin to do things.

Everyone who has had the opportunity of studying the varying dispositions of children, interesting himself in them and in their future from the earliest years on to adolescence, experimenting with new methods, finally adopts the only principle which should control any method of child education: the portioning out of instruction into various elements, each of which is more particularly intended to be taught at a definite period of the child's physical development.

When the child has reached the age of seven, eight or nine, his mother decides that the time has come for him to begin the study of music. The reasons which frequently determine her decision may be one of the following: (1) The piano is spoiling, now is a chance of keeping it in tune. (2) We have no piano, father will now decide to buy one; it will look so well in the drawing-room. (3) The child is becoming too troublesome and exuberant: playing a piano will calm him down. (4) The girl next door has begun to take lessons: my child must not be outshone by her! It is deserving of note that each of these reasons is closely linked with the idea of piano (a stringed instrument with keyboard, upright or grand, once called pianoforte because it was played sometimes *forte* and sometimes *piano* but nowadays simply called *piano* because it is always played *fortissimo*!). It never enters the mind of most parents to induce their children to take up the violin, flute, or 'cello, except when an older member of the family is already a pianist, when means do not permit of purchasing an instrument, or when some friend, who has heard Thibaut and Casals, recommends that a stringed instrument be chosen. If the parents do not come under any of these influences, they choose the piano, for the word music is inseparable from the word piano, in the minds of ninety-nine people out of every hundred.

Are we to criticise the predilection of parents for this

instrument? Not at all. The piano is an admirable instrument, the only one capable of affording complete musical sensations. It is to music what engraving – and sometimes photography – is to Nature. It expresses all harmonies and interprets approximately the most complex polyphonies. It is self-sufficing, the instrument *par excellence* of sensibility and the diffusion of musical knowledge. Mothers are right when they advise their children to take up its study, and piano teachers render the most signal service to musical art. But where mothers make a great mistake is in allowing the child to sit down at the keyboard before he either knows, understands, or loves music. For we must not count the lessons in theory which he is made to take simultaneously with his instrumental studies and during which it is imagined that there can be instilled into him in brief formulæ the very essence and ground principles of an art with whose external effects alone he is acquainted.

The first word a child utters is 'dada' or 'mamma'; this he says with pleasure and from necessity, for he knows the person corresponding to the name; he knows his father because he has seen him often and understands his *raison d'être*. It would surely be ridiculous to expect him, from early childhood, to pronounce such a word as 'municipality.' It is equally ridiculous to explain terms like syncopation or *appoggiatura* before he has become quite familiarised with their use. Musical theory is too often the study of the *signs* of music, instead of being the experience and analysis of music itself. It ought to be a consequence, not an end in itself. On the other hand, in most conservatoires, the so-called solfège classes are after all but classes in sight-reading. The pupils learn to read easily in every key (this after all is indispensable), but they do not learn to listen to music, to become more one with it. The principle I should like to develop is that "*the study of the* *piano, an instrument of musical expression, should begin only when the child has become capable of experiencing musical sensations, when he feels the desire to express them, when he has learned to analyse sensations and co-ordinate them logically."* *

A child's fingers are called upon to produce sounds and combinations of sounds mechanically, but before this his ear should be completely familiarised with these sounds, for the ear has to control the fingers. He must phrase and shade the sounds musically by means of his fingers: therefore he should know thoroughly beforehand and have experienced what a phrase is, what tone-shading is, and why it is necessary. By means of the fingers, modulations, harmonies and melodies will manifest themselves: the child should have been made aware in ear and brain of the tonal modifications created by the modulations and the physiological differences which characterise the many chords, and have known something of polyphony. The fingers have to accent certain notes metrically or emotionally, to glide softly over certain keys: consequently the child, by means of muscular contractions and relaxations, should have been enabled physically to experience the varying effects of accent. His fingers and wrists must be alternately light and heavy, active and passive, supple and rigid: and so the child should be capable of sensing throughout his body the many shades of intensity and touch.

What is contained in the exercises, the studies and the piano pieces which the child is made to play from the very beginning? Music, *i.e.* melody, harmony, counterpoint, modulation, shading, phrasing, rhythm, and also, perhaps, a little joy, a touch of sadness? What does the child know when he undertakes the interpretation of so many different elements? Frequently, alas, nothing but notes and signs. Of music itself he knows and thinks nothing: he can

* See "Rhythm in Musical Education," p. 113.

neither thrill, nor listen, nor hear aright. He can neither feel nor recognise. His very fingers have not been trained by preparatory gymnastics to take up practical study. And it is under such conditions that he will have to familiarise himself with the most abstract of all arts – that art which springs directly from the soul and appeals directly to it. Not for a moment does he dream that the soul which would apprehend and express music, must also, as William James said, "have ears"! If the ear does not catch the sounds, how can the soul be caught by musical sensations? The ear is the great controller of sounds, appreciation of which is at the foundation of all musical study. If study of the piano is capable of developing the ear, then, maybe, it should be commenced at a very early age. It is my conviction, however, that not only does this study not develop the sense of hearing, it even compromises its possibilities of improvement.

In piano playing, the production of the sounds results from the hammers striking the strings, and the various shades of expression are determined by the different ways of striking the keys.

Let a fairly heavy object strike the key corresponding to A. Whether it be the cat walking on the keyboard, the maid dusting it, or a little girl playing with one finger, the result is identically the same: the sound A will be heard. The object that fell – cat, maid, or girl – might, with the pride of the ass that played the flute in the fable, exclaim: "I, too, play the piano!"; but none of these interesting personalities can say: "I am a musician," if they cannot recognise the note as A without having seen the key that was depressed. Even if the little girl (or the cat) were to lower the key A a thousand times in succession, roughly or gently, lightly or heavily, she would be no more advanced, from the musical point of view, than a girl typist becomes literary by striking some particular key for producing the letter *b*.

The production of the sound on the piano is totally independent of the hearing faculty. The hand becomes accustomed to the various movements and skips on the keyboard, the fingers become accustomed to the action they give to the keys corresponding to the written notes, the mind may even acquire the habit of rapid analysis and the touch give effect to such advanced physical sensibility that it is possible for a pianist, with his eyes closed, to name the rapidly-executed notes played by his fingers simply by mentally following the accompanying movements. But in the case of such as are not musical or have been badly taught, *the ear is not appealed to in judging sounds*. It takes in the sound without having made any effort to call it forth, and also without having to decide whether it is correct or not. The fact that the sound is produced mechanically by the impact of the fingers, and that the only means of checking its place in the scale of sound is supplied by the *eyes* first, and afterwards by the *touch*, induces such habits of laziness as regards the ear that if the child, apart from his piano studies, does not have exercises in hearing, he will be no more advanced from the hearing point of view after twenty years than after a single month's lessons. Doubtless the production of sounds on a stringed instrument requires of the ear a slight effort which is not called for on the keyboard, but the hand of the violinist rapidly acquires the habit of placing itself on the string at the requisite height for obtaining the correct note. Doubtless also the movements of the arm are calculated – more than are the movements of the fingers – to further the development of the rhythmic sense, but taking everything into consideration, our remarks apply as much to the study of string instruments as to that of the pianoforte.

The ear can develop only when it is given something to do in distinguishing one note from another, and when, by appropriate exercises, it is enabled to determine the position of other notes, in relation to a given note, or that of chords in relation to a given chord. Out of ten pupils between seventeen and twenty years of age who play Beethoven and Chopin "with feeling" – as sentimental mothers say – if there are two who, without looking, can name the notes played by another pianist, it is because they possess *absolute pitch*, *i.e.* the rare faculty of instinctively giving the right name to every note heard. This faculty, unless it be exercised and placed at the service of the other musical powers, gives but slight superiority to its owner; but if a series of special studies can be followed, it leads to results of the most extraordinary character. Now, from the very moment of beginning to study the piano, pupils with naturally good hearing find that it gradually deteriorates. For there is nothing in these studies that calls for the collaboration of the ear, and it is well known that any physical faculty not exercised during the period of growth is checked or retarded in its development. The child best endowed physically for any kind of exercise will lose his strength and suppleness if he remains stretched on a sofa in his youth, or only breathes the open air from a motor-car. It is the same with piano practice; unless this is accompanied with exercises in hearing, it produces idleness – inertia – of the powers of hearing.

And yet, almost everything in music depends on the hearing apparatus. If the pupil cannot distinguish one note from another, he has to go through life without being able to invent successions of chords, or to transpose them, except by means of mathematical calculations which have no affinity with the living essence of music. He will stop short when playing a piece of music if his finger memory happens to fail him, for his lack of ear will prevent him from mentally reconstructing the chords and harmonies, and then passing them on to his fingers. He will never be able to grasp or interpret polyphonic works intelligently, for his lack of ear, which prevents him from mentally following the trend of a melody, will only the more certainly prevent him from grasping the simultaneous progress of several different melodies. In another direction, his finger technique will itself suffer from the lack of delicacy and exercise of his hearing apparatus, since the art of rhythm, of accenting and tone-shading, depends as much on the ear as on the touch.

The ear which controls the sounds also controls the endless varieties of sound-production; and the subtle art of combining different touches in interpretation will be a dead letter for the pupil unless his sense of hearing acts directly upon his fingers, unless there exists intimate and immediate correspondence between cause and effect, producing the artistic result required.

Certain amateur pianists shrug their shoulders or smile whenever mention is made of the pianola. Let them not forget, however, that playing scales with one's fingers on a keyboard is in itself neither more musical nor more artistic than the mechanical production of sounds on the pianola. Now, piano studies, as too often practised by non-musical pupils, seem to have no other aim than to improve the dexterity of the fingers; this is proved by the fact that the pieces for examination and competition are so frequently chosen from those which contain speed passages, not from those that call for musical ability, taste and style. . . . The "Bunte Blätter" of Schumann, the "Bagatelles" of Beethoven, the slow "Preludes" and "Nocturnes" of Chopin are considered too easy. And Haydn and Mozart are now played only by small children; they do not give sufficient scope for virtuosity! This

latter consideration governs all else in the study programme; it ranks higher than style and phrasing: to be a
good pianist is to have rapid fingers.

All the *tours de force* performed by concert performers
are obtained from young pianists; they are not expected
to be able to modulate or to transpose, to keep in rhythm,
to phrase, or to shade their tone by themselves. They
cannot therefore dispense with the music score – where
everything, as on the pianola, is noted and emphasised:
pace, nuance, breathing, all that the musically gifted pupil
should and could give effect to unaided, all that constitutes art, style, feeling: in a word, musical ability.
And why is this? Because a piano teacher cannot develop
both the virtuosity and the musical ability of a pupil.
Before becoming a virtuoso, one must be a musician.

The taste for the beautiful may be latent in the child,
but this taste will develop only if he is made acquainted
with the beautiful in all its aspects, if it is made possible
for him to analyse its proportions, to recognise its substance and become imbued with its essence. The child
loves well only that which he knows well. His first love
is that for his mother, and this love develops in proportion
as he learns to know her better, to value her unfailing
affection, her tender solicitude. In her he loves the life
that she has passed on to him, the love that she awakens
in him, and those throbbing rhythms that link together
two organisms: he loves his mother because he knows her
and recognises himself in her. And in like fashion he
learns to value every element of beauty with which he is
patiently familiarised, with all of whose peculiarities he is
made acquainted and which is thoroughly explained to
him when he asks questions.

When he begins to practise scales, will he love the
piano for itself? No, rather will he love it for the music

which it is capable of producing, those delightful sounds he has heard produced by others and which he too would like to make. Then he is seated before the keyboard, and he boldly attacks the scales and five-finger exercises, etc. But only so much of music is explained to him as concerns his fingers. If he finds the exercises wearisome, he is told to "do them, all the same: they are good for you." If he asks why they are good for him, the answer comes: "You will find out later." If his particular studies seem to him deadly dull, he is told: "You shall play good music later on." If he asks why he should play *forte* or *piano*, or why he must go slower or faster, he is told: "You will feel it in yourself later on." And so on, always later on, later on, *i.e.* when you have acquired the necessary technique, and the mechanism of it all has moulded your soul; later on, when you have lost the capacity of fresh impressions and high enthusiasms; when your ear is no longer capable of developing; when other occupations leave you no time to assimilate the elements of musical beauty . . . later on, later on! Should not mothers rather say to their children, Soon, soon, as soon as possible?

You love your children, mothers, and wish them well; but do believe me when I say, at the risk of offending you, that in sincerely desiring their good you do them ill. Some of you say: "I am so annoyed! My child does not like music; he will not practise his scales!" . . . Say, rather, that he is fond of music, whatever you may think, and that it is the scales he does not like, because he does not know the object of practising them. "And yet," you add, "little Dolly willingly practises her scales several times a day; so she must be fond of music." By no means. Dolly, impelled by that instinct of emulation and rivalry which develops so speedily in children – frequently due to the influence of parents – simply wishes to do her

scales as well as – or better than – little Margaret. And
Margaret herself likes to practise her scales only because
her mind is idle, and her piano exercises exempt her from
the exercise of her own thought. – Your child will like to
practise his scales when he knows that each of them is
different from the rest and is but a means of fixing the
keys; he will like them when his master, after asking him
to play the scale of A flat, demands "The Keel Row,"
first, in the same key, and then in another, and he feels the
different impressions produced by the two keys.

Are you aware that when the teacher plays any chance
scale to young pianists, who have conscientiously practised
all the fingerings, they scarcely ever know what scale has
been played? When he says: "I am playing Haydn's
Sonata in E major," in all probability your child experiences no tonal sensation whatsoever; and the designation,
E major, represents only words instead of awakening a
mental response. How can you expect that children so
imperfectly acquainted with the keys and the scales representing them should take pleasure in practice?

Pianoforte practice, undertaken without a certain aural
culture, utterly oppresses the individuality and does away
with the spirit of enquiry. The duty of a pedagogue is to
teach children to become – and to remain – themselves.
Like a doctor, he should mould and fashion the small
minds, make them alert and supple, instil in them the
desire to know the wherefore of things, answer all their
questions and invite them to ask others. Routine piano
practice accustoms one to the mechanical aspect of study;
the pupil copies and imitates, and ends by no longer thinking of requesting explanations. If a school inspector,
somewhat scrupulous, asks the pupils the meaning of
certain Italian words, such as *stringendo, calando*, etc.,
most of the young pianists, who are continually coming
across these expressions, are forced to answer that they do

not know their precise meaning. "Like a water-spout (*trombe*)" was the impression conveyed to the mind of a certain maiden, as she furiously pounded the keys on reaching a passage marked: *quasi tromba*!

"You preach to those already converted," will be the answer of many a music master and mistress. "We would gladly explain music to the children, playing fine passages to them and inspiring in them a love of the art, but we have not the time. The parents are continually urging us on, for they want immediate results. We barely succeed in giving their children a proper technique." "No one has the right to blame you," will be my answer. "You do what you are called upon to do. Though you feel the need of developing the child's musical ability, you are given no more than the time to develop his fingers. It is not your fault, you are simply martyrs of routine, and I shall win the approval of you all when I say: 'If children are to become musicians, their pianoforte studies should be preceded by at least two or three years' elementary study of music, including singing and exercises for ear, brain, arms, hands, feet, legs, chest, and fingers – in a word, exercises in which both physical and intellectual powers will be directed simultaneously towards the end to be attained, namely, the complete knowledge of music and its elements, and the gaining of an inner musical sense.' When children have done this, they will begin to study the piano, and then . . . you will soon have something worth reporting!"

It may be that you wonder what exercises of hands and legs have to do with music? Their aim is to arouse those spontaneous rhythms which ensure the physical and intellectual life of your child, to enable him to acquire the true notion of division of time into equal parts, and to strengthen in him the instinct of corporal balance, of proportionate movements, of rapid response to musical signs, of graded accentuations unhesitatingly obedient to the will, in a word, to perfect in him the sense of rhythm.

These studies will last two years, and the child will begin them, through play, at the age of five or six.

No one would imagine how seldom the child's sense of metre is found accompanying the sense of rhythm! Try to get your child of four to keep time in moving his legs, by counting *one*, *two*, and accenting now the *one*, now the *two*. You will be amazed to discover that the child is not master of his own movements, that neither hands nor arms are obedient to his will! The same thing happens also in almost all children of five. At six, seven and eight years, the natural instinct develops in some of them, but at least seventy-five per cent are still incapable of rhythmically accenting rapid or slow combinations of alternate movements of the limbs. . . . To think that it is at this age that they are seated in front of a piano in order to play rhythmic music with feeble little fingers, the only instruments at their disposal for rhythmic expression! When one considers also that, even in children naturally gifted rhythmically, the period between twelve and fourteen years is a critical one when co-ordination of bodily movements becomes less natural, when equilibrium of the limbs is momentarily compromised, what wonder that so few pupils play rhythmically, or even keep time at all!

Rhythmical feeling depends on psycho-physical balance; all who are badly organised rhythmically are awkward and clumsy in bodily gesture and movement, even if the ear is musical. Those who are nervous beat time in irregular jerky fashion. Lymphatic people dwell on the last note of each bar; those of sanguine disposition skip it altogether. It is possible to recognise the rhythmic powers of the orchestral conductor by his manner of presenting himself and of bowing, even before he has raised his baton. An attentive and observant master will recognise the temperament of his new pupils simply by their gait, their mode of walking and sitting. Those with easy natural gait, whose *tempo* is readily modifiable, possess in germ the suppleness of rhythm. Those who are stiff and unnatural may have an idea of metre, but their rhythmical accentuation will be sharp and peremptory. Those of irregular gait and gesture will manifest an uneasy restless rhythm. All these defects, however, may – and should – disappear, or at least be considerably lessened, by means of special exercises, arranged for the purpose of enabling the child to control all his muscles rapidly and to co-ordinate the most varied and diverse movements. Excessive resistance in the muscles of calf, hips or back, or even languid decontraction in the diaphragm, may, in a series of movements, be the cause of sudden involuntary starts which they cannot help, that is, of a lack of continuity in rhythm, or of too rapid movements, equivalent to musical note-values that are too short. For arrested attitudes, as well as the gestures which link them together, cannot take place in the right proportions of time and space unless these proportions also exist in the supple functioning – now simultaneous, now consecutive – of some group of muscles and of their opposites. On the other hand, lack of spontaneous correspondence between the pupil's will and the functioning of certain of his muscles may occasion movements too slow, *i.e.* over-prolonged musical note-values and – in the more complicated movements – rhythmic gestures without order or cohesion. Experience shows that metre itself is impeded by too slow a transmission of the will to the performing limbs.

Consequently we are justified in getting children, before they begin to study an instrument, to go through exercises intended to make their limbs, as well as the whole body, strong and supple. Then, once the bodily functions are well balanced, there will begin the study of the graphic signs corresponding to the note-values, easily expressed, no longer as on the piano by weak little fingers, but by the body as a whole, all the muscles functioning in turn or simultaneously, and communicating to the brain the rhythms of their vibrations. Thus rhythm becomes a natural corporal function sharing in the life of the individual himself. Rhythm is life. In the fine arts, rhythmic movement gives the thrills both of natural and of human life their due proportion and balance; in music, it marks the division of phrases by breathing-places, and that of beats by accents – both metrical and expressive or emotional, neither of which must interfere with the other. And so rhythm creates order in the unconscious manifestations of the individual, whilst forcing metre to become supple, and to accompany all the rhythmic swing and flow of individual life.

Each movement or series of bodily movements corresponds to a note-value or group of note-values, so that if the master teaches, together with the movement, the traditional musical sign which expresses it graphically: crotchet, semibreve, minim, etc., at the end of two years the child will easily have learned all the usual metrical notational signs, and will be capable of experiencing the sensations of time and energy which the sight of them calls up, as well as of interpreting them either plastically by gesture or musically by the voice, for naturally the voice should be used in these early studies, interpreting in easy melodies the various rhythms to be studied.

At the age of seven or eight the child will have learnt time and the fundamental laws of rhythm, without even suspecting that he has been taking lessons in music, but with increasing enjoyment, for he loves everything related to movement. Gymnastic exercises will have made him stronger and more supple. Even his voice will have developed, for naturally the master will have taught him to set the pulmonary muscles functioning. Rhythmic exercises in breathing will have broadened his chest, strengthened his lungs and doubled his powers of inspiration and expiration. If a child utterly devoid of rhythm does not obtain from these two years of musical gymnastics any appreciable immediate benefit as regards interpretation, at all events the lessons will have procured for him good health, a sensitive organism, and a clear orderly mind. The normally endowed children, whilst studying music without suspecting the fact, will also have profited by these physiological exercises.

These gymnastics, indeed, will have had a threefold object: (1) to develop the muscles, (2) to strengthen the nervous system, (3) to make the motor system an instrument with many registers, obedient alike to reason and to natural impulse, ready to vibrate in tune with music and, supple and strong – like a well-trained orchestra – ready to place itself at the service of musical art. It will also prepare the pupils directly for playing the piano, as it includes a number of exercises for fingers, wrists and arms.

And now the child, aged from seven to eight, acquainted with measure and time and the signs which express them graphically, begins to study scales and keys. Here we are dealing with musical sounds, the hearing faculties are now to begin their role. There can be no hesitation as to the means to be employed. There is one that is quite indispensable – and that is evidently why no one uses it! This consists in making the child appreciate the difference between the tone and the semitone by getting him to compare the scales with one another. The pianist is acquainted with but one scale which always proceeds from tonic to tonic and which he transposes into the different keys; he distinguishes these transpositions from one another by the different fingerings used to interpret them. All who play the piano may prove this by noting that when they are requested to think of some scale – say, the scale of A flat – the name of this scale arouses in them manual – not aural – sensations (*i.e.* they think of the second finger placed on the A flat, the third which plays the B flat, and then the C played by the thumb, etc.).

This failing may be noticed in all who have studied harmony by beginning with the piano; this apparently insignificant fact is a crushing condemnation of premature instrumental musical instruction. No sooner does the sense of musical sounds become a solely tactile sensation, unrelated to aural sensations, than all progress becomes impossible, unless a supreme effort be made to return to a natural aural appreciation. In the lessons I recommend for aural development, the child will exercise his ear without the aid of any other instrument than the voice, and it will be for the teacher to get him to hear and appreciate, first the sound of certain fundamental intervals, the octave and the fifth, then the succession of tones and semitones in the various keys, and finally the successions of the keys themselves.

Clearly the best system is to have the scales sung, not always from tonic to tonic – for in this case the tones and half-tones always follow in the same order – but from a given fixed note (suppose we take the C) which will serve as starting-point for all the scales. Then, after hearing the scale of C major several times, listen to the following succession of notes: C, D, E, F♯, G, A, B, C. . . . Do you not immediately see that it is no longer the scale of C that is being sung, that the arrangement of tones and semitones is modified, and that only the restoration of the traditional order: two tones, one semitone, three tones, one semitone, is needed to obtain the key of G major? This the children learn in a few months' lessons.

After this has come about, we may have every confidence in the future; we are certain that the ultimate functions of the ear will improve, that the children will gradually acquire relative and natural pitch, provided that the piano is not introduced before the end of the preparatory studies, in which case the final result will be endangered, for a few months of pianoforte exercises worked at too soon, *i.e.* before the ear is fully developed, suffice to obliterate the progress so far attained.

I said that the sounds will be uttered by the voice. As in this way the utterance and the perception of the sounds both take place in the head, the inevitable result is a series of close relations between the creative and receptive apparatuses of sound vibrations, and the advance towards perfection of the one will be in direct ratio to that of the other. Besides, song has many advantages over pianoforte study in the early musical education of childhood. From the physical point of view, it is proved that the child's position at the piano is bad for his bodily development unless it is ordered and adjusted in the strictest fashion from the outset: three out of every four pupils are bent-shouldered and hollow-chested. On the other hand, the vibrations of the instrument have an evil influence on the nervous system. So many cases of stomach and kidney complaints are to be found in young pianists, whereas singing develops the lungs, broadens the chest, straightens the shoulders and increases the circulation of the blood.

Of course the breathing exercises carried on during the first period of rhythmic instruction should be continued during the second, that of the study of sounds. At the first lesson in solfège, ask the pupils to take a deep breath. You will find that, for the most part, they breathe in above the ribs, causing the shoulders to rise, and lengthening, whilst at the same time narrowing, the thoracic cavity. Breathing exercises bring into play all the muscles of the trunk. The free play of the muscles of the thorax sets functioning those of the larynx, and anyone who can take a deep breath, retain it long in the chest, and exhale it within the right period of time, never sings from the throat, and very seldom with a nasal twang. There is also a fullness about his voice which vocal exercises alone could never give him. All our singing masters bewail in their pupils a number of faults which they frequently have not the time to correct. Do not these come from bad habits acquired in early childhood? How many tired and broken voices we hear, because in the singing lessons at school the children have been allowed to reach too high a chest note. When this has happened, certain professors recommend a few months' or a year's rest. But is not this remedy worse than the evil? Is suppleness and strength restored to a tired limb by keeping it motionless for weeks together? No, indeed, singing is not sufficiently cultivated either at school or in music academies. Goethe, in "Wilhelm Meister's Wander Years," traces out an ideal plan of education, containing the wisest counsels; he declares that in the first phase of education it is singing that should be the foundation of the child's physical, moral and spiritual development. And in another place he says: "Singing is the most important element in the education of a child; it is above all others!"

From the sole point of view of musical development, the practice of singing offers, in addition to the above advantages, that of subsequently supplying good interpreters in our mixed choral societies. The conductors well know that, once piano practice has begun, the pupil finds it extremely difficult to sing at sight. The fact that a young pianist can faultlessly play at sight a very difficult piece is by no means the sign of exclusively musical ability. Good sight-playing is indeed a matter of rapidity of vision and effective correspondence between the organs of transmission. The same pianist, though a good reader, will perhaps be incapable of singing even a very simple air without mistakes (I am not referring to conservatoires for professionals such as those of Paris, Brussels, etc., to which only born musicians are admitted). The fact remains that, after a certain age, it becomes exceedingly difficult for a pianist to learn to sing at sight; the ear no longer controls the voice, and it is too late to set up immediate correlation between the sight of the note to be produced and the desire to contract or to relax the vocal chords.

This is not so in the case of a child taken at an early age. If neither voice nor ear is affected, if the sense of rhythm is not absent, he inevitably succeeds after four or five years in singing at sight the most difficult airs with the utmost ease. But do not forget that the one indispensable condition is that he should not begin his instrumental studies too soon.

It may be interesting to mention an experiment I made in a large music school. Twelve children were chosen of like musical ability, *i.e.* they all had the same aptitude for recognising sounds. Six of them began to study the piano, without any other musical preparation, whilst the other six were subjected to training whose object was solely to develop their powers of ear and rhythm. At the end of a year, these latter began to study the piano, without giving up their studies of solfège, whilst the first six continued their instrumental instruction without specially cultivating the ear. Now, at the end of the second year, the six solfège pupils found themselves, from the instrumental point of view, at the same level as their companions, though they had worked at the piano only for a year — whereas the hearing faculties of the first six pianists proved to have diminished considerably.

It is impossible here to enter into details, suffice it to say that all the tonal elements of music may be studied at the outset by the sole means of that international melody called the scale. Chords, counterpoint, modulation, design and form: all is contained in this melody and may be explained by it. . . . There remains the study of tone-shading and phrasing – which, though not to be found on any programme, constitutes the best preparation for refining musical taste and developing the sense of artistic beauty. Whereas the teaching of the piano does away with the reasons for shading and accent, that of the principles of phrasing and expression creates in the pupils the sense of personal interpretation and that of the oppositions and contrasts of sound, primordial elements of musical style. This is the most important part of the teaching. The child possesses an innate sense of beauty; he is passionately interested in everything that reveals to him new and unsuspected beauties. He also likes to know the reasons of things, frequently taking his toys to pieces to find out what there is in them. The many indications throughout a piece of music really explain too much. He gives effect to what is marked, plays *forte* or *piano*, slowly or rapidly, *because it is all written down*. No personal artistic concern enters into his interpretation, nor is there any effective play for his creative instinct. But what a pleasure it would be if he knew the easy and logical principles of phrasing and expression,* if he could read a melody free from all annotation, interpreting it as he pleased and guided solely by his general knowledge of the principles of beauty, *i.e.* of the laws that govern movements, set up contrasts and balance periods.

In this he succeeds very easily, for there is nothing to oppose his progress. He is confronted with the music

* Formulated by Mathis Lussy in his ingenious *Musical Expression* (Novello).

alone and is daily conscious of an inner growth and development. During the long and uninterrupted course of
his studies, he has used nothing but his own natural
ability; his muscles, now supple and strong, are the
eager ministers of his will; he can produce rhythmic and
well-accented music.   His ear has been accustomed to
distinguish the various sounds; he can listen to, perceive,
and analyse their progressions and correlations.   His
voice has been trained by progressive exercises; guided by
a well-trained ear, he can control the sounds produced by
his fingers, interpret and even create little melodies which
he sings heartily and in which his personality already
begins to assert itself. In a word, he has become a
musician, capable of appreciating the elements of music and
eager for new musical sensations. Then you may allow
him to study instrumental technique; it will be a joy for
him to practise scales and exercises, for he will understand
what he is doing and how the sounds are linked together.
He will transpose, prelude and improvise naturally and
easily, without feeling his way; and he will make rapid
progress in the mechanical element of his work, for his
fingers, already trained by rhythmic gymnastics, will
become the interpreters of alert and vibrant thought.
The well-taught child is extremely fond of improvisation,
for it exercises his innate powers of expression and
creation. He who is able to express himself succeeds all
the sooner in expressing the feelings of others.

   The results just mentioned are not illusory; they were
obtained over three centuries ago in the Flemish and
Italian *scholæ*. Any normally-gifted child should obtain
them without difficulty. But even if, from among the
children taught after this fashion there are a few who make
no progress owing to an utter lack of ability, one great
advantage will have been gained: both masters and
parents will know where they stand. Unmusical children

need no longer study any instrument, and both music and society at large will be the gainers. The world is flooded with mediocre and incapable players who have studied an instrument without loving it, continue listlessly to practise so as not to lose the money expended on their studies, and bore themselves and everybody within hearing. If some mothers object that such a musical programme is a very long one, that the ordinary school programme is already well filled, and that they do not wish to make artists, but only amateurs, of their children . . . then my reply is that present-day pianoforte instruction in no way meets their desires, for it tends – even if applied to amateurs – to create virtuosi and requires a vast amount of study from the pupils. The instruction I advise is far shorter and less fatiguing, it is most suitable for "amateurs" from the fact that it will make them "love" music. Two to three hours' daily practising of scales and arpeggios, or three-quarters of an hour devoted to becoming musicians: choose which is the more useful, the more humanly artistic. And if you wish your children to become virtuosi, all the more reason to develop their musical ability at an early age, for there is nothing in the world more obnoxious or grotesque than a virtuoso devoid of the soul of music.

Then there are the children who have begun the piano and have already mastered their instrument. What are they to do? Is it possible further to develop their faculties of hearing and of rhythm? I believe it is, but they will need much determination and perseverance. They will have to trample their pride under foot and become persuaded that everything their piano has taught them does not belong wholly to the realm of pure music but constitutes simply a musical substitute, that their interpretation of a piece of music is for the most part quite mechanical and not dictated by individuality of temperament, mature judgment, a firmly established instinct and a truly artistic sensibility.

This conscientious self-examination and obstinate search after truth athwart paths of pedantry will assuredly, at some time of their career, be made by sincere and independent pupils who, sooner or later, discover what they lack and then, by hard work, seek to acquire that knowledge which their reason judges indispensable for their full development. But alas, what becomes of the rest, feeble and unaware of their condition, whose parents do not feel the necessity for a complete artistic course, who are content with a few outward results and sacrifice the future of their children without any suspicion of the irreparable wrong they are doing them? As a rule, is it not the parents themselves who prevent their children from doing their preparatory work slowly, and with assiduity and confidence? The fact of seeing them spend two or three years in perfecting their sense of hearing, the results of which are not immediate and do not call forth the applause of friends and acquaintances at family gatherings, seems as though it must detract from the ability of their children. Occasionally they consent to the child trying a new education for twelve months, then they stop the lessons under one pretext or another. So many children say to their solfège master: "I should like to continue, but mother will not let me." – "Why will she not let you?" – "It takes too much time, and I have other lessons." – "And are you giving up the piano too?" – "Oh, no, sir!" . . . No, indeed, there is no giving up the piano. The piano, in spite of all reasoning, is music; it is sacred Art. The piano is taboo! It is worshipped as the golden calf; to it are sacrificed common sense, the higher musical delights, natural sensibility, good taste, and even the very health of the children. It may be that the parents have not been warned, that they are not aware of their lack of foresight.

Leave the piano in the background for a certain

period and let your child resume the study of the two essential elements of music: rhythm and sound. Hand him over to trained masters who will teach him rightly to co-ordinate his movements, to call upon a will power which rapidly and unhesitatingly controls his whole body, to count the time mentally, to attack a musical phrase on any beat of the bar, to end it without a hitch, to play slow or fast without affectation, to accent the right note, to mould the phrase, as it were, with the requisite energy and suppleness. The beneficent effect of rhythmic gymnastic exercises will counteract the disastrous influence of the piano from the point of view of nerves, in so many young girl students. It is always possible to make progress in the development of the ear if one has the will and is able to continue to exercise it. It is never too late to do the right thing! And the result will compensate persevering and conscientious pupils for the effort expended. Instead of putting up with music, they will adapt their temperament to it, they will appreciate and love it in their own persons.

Pianoforte teachers will find a longer musical preparation in instrumental studies to their advantage. All their observations on style and interpretation will bear fruit. The pupils will of their own accord avoid gross faults that would shock a musical sense which is now more refined. There will no longer be the risk of having studies stopped half-way, for teachers will have as pupils only those whose musical talent has been tested by the right preliminary tasks. The parents too will have every reason for self-congratulation, for they will no longer have to tolerate the painful sounds usual at the beginning of a child's practice. Will they not be pleased to hear their sons and daughters interpret classical and modern works with taste and appreciation, to find that they can play by ear or improvise perfectly-balanced melodies, accompany songs in any key, arrange an air for chorus, and even play for dancing? In a word, will they not be glad to find that they enter into a closer relationship with art by bringing it into everyday life, thanks to a logical system of training which places the body under control of the mind, which latter it initiates into a profound acquaintance with beauty, and all its fruitful and regenerative influences?

VIII

EURHYTHMICS AND THE EDUCATION
OF THE BLIND

THOSE interested in education are concerned at the large
numbers, who for one cause or another have lost the use
of their organs of sight and hearing. A host of scientists
have dealt with the re-education of atrophied or mutilated
limbs, and have performed wonders in the art of restoring
the natural powers of movement or of substituting artificial aids, but no attempts at sense re-education appear to
have been made with a view to supplementing the loss of
sight or hearing, by reason of other methods employed in
the education of the blind and deaf. These methods,
nevertheless, would appear susceptible of improvement,
and the special studies and experiments we have made in
Geneva afford us the hope that soon an improvement will
take place in the distressful condition of so many human
beings deprived for ever of the full use of their faculties.
Our experiments are perhaps too recent to supply definite
conclusions; still, we think they are calculated to interest
those who seek to "repair the irreparable," and also to
direct some of us along fresh paths of progress.

When visiting schools for the blind, I had always been
impressed by the weak constitution, the physical awkward-
ness, the lack of balance or poise, the nervousness and
apparent inattention of most of the children. The masters
were all agreed in attributing their awkward attitudes,
inertia of facial expression and dislike of moving about, to
their lack of self-confidence, their dread of not being

appreciated, of not knowing what people were thinking of them, of their incapability of complete self-expression. Whereas normal children read in the faces of their teachers an ever-present solicitude and interest, blind children cannot constantly ascertain that they are not being neglected, when they are not spoken to. During a silence, whether short or prolonged, they imagine themselves forgotten and gradually assume the habits and aspect of the lonely individual, the sombre air of detachment and abandonment seen in the prisoner. Their doctors have often told me how difficult it is, when they fall ill, to convince them of the necessity of asserting themselves to resist the disease and so hasten their cure. Their powers of moral and physical resistance are frequently inadequate, and few seem to care greatly about living.

Nevertheless, on several occasion I had the opportunity – while watching blind children listening to music – of finding on many a little face a sort of furtive interest, budding smiles and nascent energies. And on discovering also that the majority of them receive no more lessons in music or gymnastics than do normal children, I wondered if a special psycho-physical education based on the study of sound and rhythm – during which the master would ever be on the look-out to rouse the attention and fix the concentration of the class, by means of the countless resources of music and the voice, and of joy in movement – might not be calculated to develop the powers of concentration of the blind, to awaken their curiosity, develop their imagination and their natural craving for expansion and expression, creation and communication with their surroundings?

While giving lessons in Eurhythmics to normal children at Hellerau, the idea came to me to ask them to go through certain exercises blindfold, in order to try and analyse the effect of the powers of vision upon the physical bearing, the concentration, the energy and the nervous condition of the children. I at once noticed that nervous subjects became far more nervous when deprived of light, that the "rash and eager" type completely lost all self-control, and that only those possessed of a calm clear intellect, together with a supple and elastic muscular system, found pleasure in the exercises and rapidly solved problems whose object was to give them definite notions of distance and direction, line and form, to strengthen their sense of space and develop their motor-tactile sense. I came to the conclusion that a systematic study of degrees of energy and time in movement and of rapid contraction and relaxation of the muscles – together with exercises that aim at increasing the number of reflex movements and harmoniously training the nervous system by alternately calming and exciting it – would prove a valuable aid in the general education of the blind.

From that time onward, my mind was engaged upon this important and complex question. Two of my pupils, Miss Meredyll of London and M. Joan Llongueras of Barcelona, undertook to introduce Eurhythmics into classes of blind pupils which I had the good fortune to visit. The results obtained were so remarkable that the educational authorities unhesitatingly favoured the continuation of these special studies. The teachers in the London school were unanimous in declaring that the children were passionately fond of their lessons and that their general deportment had greatly improved. The pupils attempted to utilise their knowledge of rhythm in their other everyday school occupations, and the doctors also noted in them greater resistance to disease. Unfortunately the classes were held only twice a week, whereas daily, even twice daily, instruction should be insisted upon. M. Llongueras also states, in the last number of

Le Rythme that his blind pupils attain "a very sure and precise notion of the space in which they move. Their movements become more definite and assured. Eurhythmics vivifies the personality, enriches their lives, develops their imagination, strengthens their will and clarifies their thinking processes. They have become bolder and more optimistic and have felt growing up within them the sense of expression, a feeling of pleasure and enthusiasm."

I too have been deeply touched during the lesson to find awakening within them, under the influence of music and of the corresponding bodily movement, a serene joy, which transfigures their poor little faces: their features seemed to glow with an inner light.

Thereupon I determined to devote closer study to this absorbingly interesting question, and to try to set up more intimate correlations between the ordinary eurhythmic exercises and the classic education of the blind. I also endeavoured to evolve new exercises more specially adapted to their physical and mental condition.

The *sense substitution*, so frequently spoken of in reference to the blind, is but a product of the defensive instinct in cases when one of the means of self-preservation happens to be lacking. This substitution comes about gradually as the result of spontaneous experiments generated by necessity; it is not – as it was once thought to be – a legitimate compensation granted by Nature to an individual deprived of one or other of the senses. With few exceptions, the tactile sensibility of the blind is no more acute than that of normal persons; neither is their keenness of hearing. There is no definite connection between the faculties of hearing, touch and smell in human beings. The reason that the blind differentiate their impressions of touch more completely than do normal persons is not due to special propensities, but to the constant practice imposed on them by circumstances, enabling them also to set up relations between their motor and tactile sensations and their sense of space. The reason that the keenness of touch of a Helen Keller or a Laura Bridgmann appears superior to that of normal people is that the intelligence of these two blind and deaf girls was above the average, and enabled them to a greater extent to conceive and attempt exercises for strengthening the qualities of their remaining senses. Thus we may take for granted that one of the first objects to be attempted by those who undertake the education of the non-seeing is to develop their *imaginative* powers and enable them to associate rapidly the greatest possible number of diverse sensations.

Some of those born blind consider that only non-seeing teachers are capable of controlling the experiments of their blind brothers, because sighted people could not place themselves in the physical and mental state necessary for attempting exercises which aim at the education of the senses. There is a basis of truth in this. Nevertheless, a blind teacher cannot possess a sighted person's faculties of *control*; the experiments of the former need to be supplemented, directed and animated by those of the latter. The explanations of the fully educated blind person will incite the normal teacher to seek after means of establishing relations between the state of blindness and that of clear vision, between the impressions produced by the muscular sensation of space and by the vision of space, between judgments dicated by the ear and those given by the eye.

On the other hand, though certain scientists (such as Griesbach and Kunz) discover that blindness frequently causes a weakening of touch, of hearing and of smell, it is my impression that this weakening is mainly due to the lack of vital resistance which may be observed in many subjects, whose lack of confidence in the reality of their existing powers produces in them a general state of debility and physical inferiority. It is of supreme importance to inform the blind child of the wealth of the resources that he has at his disposal in spite of his affliction, to replace the vision of external realities by that of inner realities, and gradually, once he has come to see clearly within himself, to induce him to make centrifugal this centripetal clear-vision, and to find for himself, under the direction of a sighted person who explains external things to him, the means of communicating in his own way with this "external" world, while escaping from himself.

One fact is certain: the sighted person is frequently prevented by the intensity of constant ocular sensations from forgetting external conditions in order to concentrate upon himself. He has at his disposal means of control that are wholly external, and he forgets to analyse — or even utilise — his muscular sensations, when it is a matter of finding his direction and regulating his bodily movements. The same experiments to which a rational education ought to subject the seeing person in order to enable him to know himself completely, ought therefore to be imposed on the blind, and in the latter case the experiments will be still more conclusive and decisive.

Once the sighted person has his eyes shut, he experiences the same physical inconvenience as does the blind, the same difficulty in performing natural and rapid gestures without contortion or grimace, in keeping balance, walking in a straight line, or finding his way in different directions. Nevertheless, after a short time, he becomes accustomed to dispense with the guiding-marks created by the eye and is conscious that his powers of directing himself depend on new muscular appreciations dictated by a special sense, which is as rich in easy natural manifestations as is the visual sense.

In a word, when you or I make our way towards a certain point in space, it is the eye, so to speak, that gives our body the desire and the initiative of movement, imposing on it the requisite orientation.* The starting-point is not in the heavy part of our limbs, though this part should act in all spontaneous movements, in all unpremeditated bodily manifestations. Our vision prevents us from gauging the true proportions of space, and, in addition, often deceives us in the matter of perspective. But when we close our eyes and are told to take twelve steps forward and then stop, our muscular consciousness gives us precise information as to the space to be traversed, and we feel ourselves in close communion with it. Similarly, the pianist becomes truly master of the expanse of the keyboard only when he can play with his eyes shut, can realise just where the key should be struck by means of the experienced relations of this spot with the extreme keys instead of requiring to be shown it by his eyes. The main thing in these studies of muscular and spatial relations is to ascertain that the blind man is sure of his steps and possesses the peace of mind which such security engenders. These studies need to be supplemented by those which aim at enabling the body to move and cease moving *without moral, intellectual or physical resistance*, and to do this at all speeds and at the right moment, without disturbance or loss of balance. It should be remembered that the normal man, not specially educated, is incapable

* Here, naturally, I am speaking of those who enjoy the free use of their limbs. The atoxic or the myclitic who have lost a part of their sensibility and space-direction find it difficult to walk although they have retained their power of vision. To restore the sense of balance in the former and increase the sensibility of the latter, there must be re-education which, in its first period, does not need the help of sight.

of taking a certain number of steps determined beforehand, without finding it extremely difficult to secure that
they are even and straight, and especially to halt at the
end of the period fixed upon. For stopping depends on
the weight of the body, and only precise education or
training can balance the oscillations of this weight and
regulate the muscular inhibitions which ensure bodily
equilibrium. To cross a room alone, with several pairs of
eyes levelled at you, is no easy matter, and general stiffness of the limbs is the frequent result of our incapacity
to walk in a reasoned manner. Now, the blind must
always reason when they move from one place to another.
Consequently, it is absolutely necessary that they should
attune their bodily mechanism to their nervous impulsions. And the exercises in starting suddenly with precision, halting, modifying the length of steps and the
lines to be followed, counting the number of steps to be
taken, etc., . . . should be combined with a constant look-
out for such starting-points as are most calculated to
ensure the exactness and harmony of the movements.
This exactness and harmony is generally compromised by
futile muscular interventions, just as over-elaborate scor-
ing will confuse the rendering of simple and natural
harmonies and melodies.

How will the teacher be able to tell the blind child of
the origin of his movements, their true starting-points,
their various degrees of dynamic force, their harmonisation and orchestration? By first explaining to him that
every movement is produced by muscular contraction and
enabling him to note both the external and the internal
effects of this contraction. To give him the sensation of
contraction, he must become accustomed to the state of
utter *relaxation*. This is very difficult, for while we often
note in the blind child a state of general weakness, certain
parts of his body such as the shoulders and the neck, for

instance, are constantly contracted. Again, the muscles of face and hands are continually twitching with nervous contractions. It is especially necessary, therefore, that the functioning of the diaphragm should be maintained by repeated exercises, and that all the other muscles should be capable of entering into – and remaining in – a state of complete rest, so that each effort of contraction, the origin of each movement, may become easily controllable. It is by touch, in the first place, by feeling the teacher's arm or leg that the blind pupil will be able to control or check the external effect of contraction. He will learn to imitate these effects on each of his own limbs, to isolate them and finally to combine and harmonise them. Some particular muscular effort is necessary for placing the arm or the whole body in some particular direction, and any effort of different nature or intensity is recognised by him as compromising the exactness of orientation. Later, I will indicate the different methods of ensuring this exactness and of definitely locating the body in its environment. These experiments will be supplemented by the study through touch of anatomical casts and of fragments of sculptures representing bodies in motion. The blind pupil will be able to recognise the external form of the movements, according as they project themselves forwards or not. Any muscular contraction modifies the gravity of a limb, and bodily equilibrium depends on an exact knowledge of the co-operating and the conflicting forces.

The obtaining of this equilibrium frees the mind from certain disturbing factors often manifested in the blind pupil by the harassed expression of his face when his body begins to move or when this movement stops. Only when conveniently seated does the non-seeing person show a countenance in calm repose. But even this tranquillity resembles too closely that of death, whereas the halt of a movement does not imply the stoppage of life. Every stop is a preparation for a resumption of activity. A study of the various modes of stopping and re-starting should form part of the education of the blind, as also of those who see. A rapid correspondence should be set up and maintained between the nervous system and the motor apparatus. And all exercises in Eurhythmics without exception are meant to produce plastic, visceral and tactile impressions which communicate life to the brain. There is nothing mysterious about this correspondence. Instead of leaving each blind person to find out for himself the laws of psycho-physical associations, it is quite simple to put him in a position to discover them rapidly and easily by explaining certain methods of orchestrating movements, which he can acquire by study far more readily than does the sighted person. Indeed, the spatial and tactile sensations of the latter are no more than a resultant, an echo and transposition of the visual sensations. From the moment that the blind man is able to control, both from within outwards and from without inwards, the many contractions of his muscles, his sense of orientation naturally becomes more acute. Indeed, if a certain contraction of the arm is recognised by him as inevitably setting this limb in a given direction, all that he has to do is to harmonise with this contraction all those which give the body the same direction, and so the body becomes aware of the space in which it moves.

The security of his movements is made very easy for the normal child through his powers of imitation. "Walk like me; do just as I do," says the master to a child uncertain in gait or gesture. The child copies, checks, corrects and becomes master of the movements he observes. The blind child should be given the same possibilities of imitation, but instead of *looking* at the master's arm moving or his fist clenching, he will *feel* this arm and wrist, and then will feel his own in order to discover the difference, and model and grade his gestures, both dynamically and geometrically, according to the tactile image offered by the master or by a more advanced pupil. Indeed, this system is used by Dr. Besse of Geneva in the restoration of patients who have lost both the stereognostic sense and that of muscular contraction and relaxation.

It is not sufficient to strengthen the muscular and spatial sense in the blind man. He must also be taught to conjecture the obstacle beforehand, to keep clear of it, and finally to surmount it. The "obstacle" sense, brilliantly analysed by Pierre Villay in his fine work, *Le Monde des Aveugles,** is constantly manifested to the normal person, when absent-mindedly crossing the street. Of a sudden he halts, *feeling* that he is confronted with a wall or a bend in the path. He becomes aware of the presence of the wall as much by sensing an obstacle to the air stream as by unconscious vision. The approach of the extremity of a path cut by a cross-street is revealed by the declivity of the soil. Once the street is crossed, the sensitive foot *feels* the approach of the new path, by reason of the modifications of the ground.

I remember, after an air raid on Paris in 1916, finding my way from the rue des Abbesses to the rue Montmartre, without moonlight or the aid of a lamp, without jostling the passers-by or knocking against the houses, simply by reason of the mysterious warnings I received from certain sensations on the forehead, stomach and limbs. When I ask a pupil to proceed blindfold down a long row of pupils touching one another and request him to make a sudden right turn to cross the row at the

---

* *Le Monde des Aveugles, essai de Psychologie,* by Pierre Villay, *agrégé de l'Université,* published by Flammarion, 26 rue Racine. The reading of this book has helped me considerably to understand both the mentality and the motor activity of the blind. – (E. J.-D.)

spot where contact is broken between two persons a yard apart it is seldom that the pupil makes a mistake, and does not feel at what spot the obstacle of the bodies is broken. Similarly, he is rarely mistaken when requested to cross an empty room and try to divine the presence of somebody in any given place. He is warned of this presence – or of this vacuum in the continuity of living obstacles – by a certain atmospheric or caloric differentiation, by modifications in floor vibrations, by hearing sound of breathing, also by certain olfactory emanations. Numerous experiments are to be – and have already been – tried in this domain; their frequent success enables us to assert their efficacy. From the purely auditory point of view – the one which concerns me most in my lessons to normal children – I can easily direct them, when, blindfold, they are requested to go to a certain spot, guided by a voice singing *pianissimo* as it moves about the room, or by the piano on which a few chords are struck, or even by the sound of the steps of a sighted pupil who must be followed as he crosses and re-crosses the room. After a very short time, walking up and down stairs becomes an easy matter. In accordance with changing plans stated beforehand, they mount three steps, descend two, again mount five, and without excessive lack of balance, modify the direction at will. Seeing the ease with which children adapt themselves to these exercises, which manifestly call for a certain knowledge of the natural displacements of the weight of the body, has often made me think of the dismay with which, in a large institute for the blind, I once saw the inmates, who had used the main staircase for several years, frequently stumble, and even fall, as they went up and down. Analytical exercises conscientiously practised for a fortnight would assuredly have enabled them to move about quite easily on those stairs.

The reason why we can confidently recommend a series

of exercises calculated to develop the sense of space and of obstacles, is that three or four exercises of this kind, gone through safely by the pupil, quickly and easily fit him for new exercises, whether similar or different: and this because of the associations of ideas created by a *muscular memory* perpetually nurtured and developed. . . . Certain physiologists class this kind of memory among the totally unconscious manifestations of the individual, and certainly he has to determine, without reasoning, con-catenations of movements that have become mechanical. This memory, however, may be developed by reasoned exercises, and then the number of associations consider-ably increases. For instance, man, when walking, links his steps two by two, and if he is asked to scan this series in regular accents, he accents without reasoning the first of a bar in duple time, but certain individuals will prefer to strike the ground with the right foot, while others will use the left. After a month of military service, a soldier is automatically reduced to the "left, right." When mov-ing from place to place, the idea never enters his head to use the right foot first. In our eurhythmic classes, march-ing in three, four, and five time, with the first beat of each series accented, very soon becomes automatic. The mere calling by the master of the number 3, 4, 5, or 6, releases the unthinking dynamic forces of the accentuation. Later on, simply on hearing the music, they will instinctively beat time; a new reflex is created. Similarly muscular appreciation of space by using an arm or leg, placed at one of the nine degrees of height or the nine surrounding planes studied in Eurhythmics, soon becomes instinctive (see diagrams Figs. 5 and 7, pp. 20 and 22). At the word of command: plane 3, degree 5, for instance, the arm automatically places itself in a determined position, and if the master asks the pupil to direct the whole of his body in the same plane, the muscles instinctively do what is necessary. Thus it is possible to supply the memory with guiding marks, to increase the number of automatic movements, to devise new reflex movements and considerably enrich the scale of motor habits as well as that of their combinations and concatenations.

Only when this rational initiation into the mechanical life of movements is ended can the education of the *temperament* of the blind pupil be undertaken and a strong and constant appeal be made to him to abandon himself confidently and unhesitatingly to his spontaneous impulses, utilising his own individual bodily rhythms. Indeed, it must not be forgotten that the sole reason for the blind pupil's apparent lack of motor rhythm is due to his ignorance of his powers of movement. If the teacher succeeds in developing confidence in the pupil's own powers, and assuring him that it is possible for him to make a few bodily movements quite safely, then his imagination will expand unchecked, his temperament will awaken and fall into tune with his character, and a more intense stream of life will fill his entire being.

One of the first principles of Eurhythmics is the elimination of useless movements. A pupil who has worked the necessary time will walk and move harmoniously, without thinking of harmony or grace of motion, but solely because he instinctively employs only the muscles needed for action; hence there is absence of conflict, a condition of permanent balance. In expressing his thoughts, his gestures will be rapid and convincing, for the person to whom they are addressed and who is to be convinced perceives no groping in space, no hesitation or muscular conflicts, whereas most speakers indulge in endless gestures, in the hope of finding one that is convincing, and give merely the impression of being agitated because they cannot find it. Thus, if things are placed without any order in the drawers of a chest, the unfortunate person looking for some particular object is compelled to open the drawers hurriedly one after another and upset their contents, his actions become increasingly numerous, hurried and feverish, his mind is agitated simultaneously with his hands, his eyes flash fire, and sometimes his trembling lips utter words he afterwards regrets. A series of calm and expressive gestures not only reveals an adequate state of mind but is also capable of restoring calm to a mind from which it is momentarily absent.

The blind man seldom gesticulates: this is owing to mistrust, not to calculation. He does not attempt to emphasise his speech by eloquent gestures because he has not been taught to search for gestures himself, and he can neither imitate nor understand the value of the eloquent gestures of others. Consequently he must remain deprived, for lack of education, not only of a sure means of communication with his surroundings, but also of the only means a man has of calming his nervous agitation by expressing it externally in a rhythmic manner. It cannot be denied that rhythmic movements possess a calming influence upon the nervous system. Most neurasthenics are people whose tempestuous desires find no means of outward expression; hence, a state of mental disorder results. From the moral point of view, would it not be very advantageous to teach the blind child many and varied mechanical movements of his body, even if this study did not enable him to employ these mechanical movements for entering into relation with the outer world? To see clear within oneself is surely one of the best methods of realising that one is clairvoyant. The development of motor association of ideas and of polyrhythmic faculties too often comes about *unconsciously* in the blind during their childhood. Would it not be well to lighten their task? Every one knows what wonderful results have been obtained by teachers in schools for the blind, how concerned and solicitous they are in the education of their pupils. In very many cases the results are wonderful.* Nevertheless it seems to me that in the domain of the tactile and motor senses their experience would need to be supplemented by numerous exercises in Eurhythmics, which indeed appear as though they had been devised for this very purpose.

I would refer the reader who wishes to make acquaintance with these exercises in detail to my works on *Rythmique* and *Plastique animée.*†

All exercises suited to the normal child, when adapted to cases of blindness, cannot fail to be equally suitable in the education of the blind. Their aim is to make the children conscious of themselves, to reveal to their body its numerous motor faculties and to increase the number of vital sensations. Simultaneously they reveal the existence of higher artistic forms, for art springs direct from the knowledge of life. By familiarising the child with life, its desires and struggles, its tumults and calms, its disorders and its harmonies, we develop in him the love of art and the desire to practise it.

The following is a list of special exercises expressly intended for the blind. Most of them have been attempted, with considerable interest and benefit, by normal children or adults blindfold. Though the list is incomplete, it gives a general idea of our system.

Exercises for Developing the Sense of Space and the Muscular Sense

1. Run or walk confidently, halt at the word of command, then backwards to the starting-point.

* In certain schools of massage for those blinded in the war the teaching was almost entirely through plastic means, with the help of anatomical casts in half-relief. † *Rhythmic Movement,* vols. I and II – Novello.

The same exercise on the steps.

2. Control of straight line, arm extended. Move about between two rows of chairs without touching them.

3. Move about in a labyrinth made up of chairs, tables, etc., the plan of which has previously been explained.

4. Rhythm of steps to be realised in a series of given spaces.

5. Walk a certain number of steps (fixed beforehand), then suddenly turn in a certain plane.

6. Kneeling without the aid of the arms, in all planes. The same with the aid of the arms, placed in some other degree.

7. Place the hands in a certain plane or degree, make them into a *fixed point*, and move the body without changing the hands' position in space.

8. Two rows of pupils facing each other. Each pupil in the first row, with outstretched arms, touches the palm of the hand of a pupil in row 2. One step backwards, then again one step forward, clapping the hand that has been released. . . . Then two steps, three steps, eight steps, twelve steps . . . etc.

9. Two rows, facing each other. Each pupil of row 1 going to his right along row 2, claps, keeping time, the hand of the first pupil opposite him, then the second, third, fourth, etc. The spaces between each pupil should be varied, as also the number of steps to be taken.

10. Blind pupils proceed hand in hand in single file, led by a sighted pupil, amid obstacles, inclined planes, etc. The attitude of the sighted pupil, his arm contracting or relaxing, his leg rising or bending, reveal to the next pupil the nature of the obstacles, and these indications are passed from one blind pupil to another.

11. The pupil walks as he pleases about the room, dropping every so many steps one of a series of objects he holds in his hands. Then he turns round and must recover

the objects by remembering the number of steps taken and their direction.

12. The pupil, having learnt to recognise the height of each of his companions by the muscular sensation of his raised arm placed on their shoulders, must move along a row formed by the rest, and recognise them by their height.

13. Two rows of pupils advance slowly to meet each other (hand stretched forward) and attempt to cross each other.

14. The pupil is set in front of objects placed at different altitudes and in planes which the master has enumerated beforehand. He must take hold of these objects one after another, then of two at once, though on different planes.

15. Throw balls to a given height, controlled by muscular sensation and the sense of duration, then catch them to certain rhythms.

16. With key in hand, walk towards a door and place the key in the lock.

17. The foot being in a certain plane, place knee or chest in another plane and walk in the right direction.

18. A sighted pupil leads a blind one in three or four planes, then the blind one goes over the ground alone.

19. A score of chairs are placed in a row, so many inches apart (the length of an average step, for example). The fifth, the ninth, etc., are separated from the next one by a greater space. The pupil mounts on to the first chair, and, leaning on a sighted pupil, walks from chair to chair, successfully stretching across the larger spaces of which he has been told beforehand.

20. The pupils are seated on chairs placed in a row. Each one rises, walks in a given plane, then returns and sits down in the chair he has left, or on that placed beside him, etc.

21. Six or eight pupils are arranged so as to represent a very simple geometrical figure. One pupil goes over the lines they form, touching them with his hand. Then he calls out the name of the figure, draws it, or – the pupils having modified their positions – attempts to put them back into their first position.

Exercises for Developing Tactile Sensibility and Muscular Consciousness

1. Realise on the arms of a sighted pupil the *crescendos* and *decrescendos* of muscular innervation, in their relation to fullness of gesture – then execute these dynamic nuances oneself. Control is easy to establish if, in moving his arms, the pupil can place the end of his finger on different steps of a ladder or on pegs planted in the wall and serving as guide-marks.

2. Determine the length of steps, the extent of lunges by the same method. Regulate body balance by means of the muscular sensation created by displacement of the weight of the body.

3. Walk slowly, leaning against a sighted pupil or one half-blind, and imitate his steps and gestures. Subsequently, the same exercise will be done without any support; contact will no longer be that of one epidermis with another, but that of two radiations.

4. (*a*) Proceed barefoot along a line of cloth, halt at each break in the line.

(*b*) Halt before an open door or an arranged draught.

(*c*) Halt before a spot – slightly perfumed – on the wall.

(*d*) Proceed with one hand against a partition made of various materials; halt at each change noticed in the nature of the partition (wood, cloth, etc.)

5. Analyse the contour of a piece of furniture or some

other object. Find this object, when included among several others.

6. Keep the muscles of the face absolutely calm, and analyse the successive or associated contractions of brow, eyelids, neck, mouth, eyebrows, with reference to the movements they create. – Associations and dissociations of shoulder movements. – It is very important to obtain control of the *facial* movements during the exercise of the other motor functions, to check any perturbation of the physiognomy, during the reactions of the other parts of the body.

7. Try to obtain a general static condition favourable to attention. Avoid contractions of the hands whilst paying attention; do not stretch out the neck in the direction of the sound, etc.

8. Stand the children in a row, with irregular intervals between some of them. The pupil passes along this row, recognising the intervals from the fact that he is aware that the stream of animal heat has been interrupted.

9. The pupil feels the entire contour of an object, then he recognises this object among several others when *only one side* of it is offered to him. The same when in front of a companion, whose brow is found after feeling his shoulder, etc.

10. A rope is outstretched and knots made at various points. After ascertaining the distance between the knots, the pupil is requested to touch the first, the second, the tenth knot, etc.

11. Walk towards a wall; stop as soon as the obstacle is felt.

12. Determine the number of marbles or other objects placed in the pupil's hand (then in both hands). Analyse the nature of the objects.

Etc., etc.

*Exercises for Developing the Auditory Faculties in their
Relation to Space and the Muscular Sense*

1. The pupils, standing anywhere in the room, guide
themselves by the voice of the master. He moves about,
uttering a sound or beating a drum from time to time;
they walk in the direction of the sound. . . . The master
plays the piano, the pupils, attracted by the sound, make
their way towards the piano, to right or left, pass round
it, retreat from it during the *decrescendo*, etc.

2. The pupils attempt to guess how many steps of a
certain length separate them from some one loudly clapping his hands.

3. The master strikes simultaneously *x* strokes on the
floor with a stick, and *y* strokes with something giving a
different sound. The pupils should recognise the number
of strokes sounded by each instrument. The same with
three instruments, also with piano and triangle, piano and
drum, triangle, drum and cymbals, etc., etc.

4. Learn to listen with *both* ears while avoiding all
contortion; analyse the sound by turning the head in all
directions.

5. Walk behind a sighted person, guided by the sound
of his steps, his words, his singing, an instrument he
plays, etc.

6. (*a*) Walk on a surface spread with cloth and analyse
the resonance of the steps. Halt when the foot strikes a
spot where the cloth is absent.

(*b*) Walk along walls covered with cloth, occasionally
uttering sung or spoken sounds and noting their resonance. Halt at the places where the cloth is missing or is
replaced by wood or some other material.

7. Pretend to be deaf, and try to perceive sound vibrations with the teeth, the bones, all the individual's sound
walls.

8. Distinguish the directions of several sounds uttered simultaneously in various parts of the room.

9. A sighted pupil runs four steps, stamping on the ground. The blind pupil joins him in eight steps (or six or ten).

10. The pupils stand in a circle. One pupil moves about in spirals round each individual, guided by the sound he makes in clapping his hands.

11. The pupils, standing in a circle, have each to sing a different sound communicated beforehand to a soloist standing in the centre. They turn in a circle; then the singing stops. The soloist has to make his way towards the pupil uttering the particular sound designated by the master.

12. Four pupils each say a different word simultaneously – or sing each a different sound. One pupil tries to differentiate these words and sounds.

13. In deep silence, a ball is thrown on to the floor; it rebounds and comes to a stop. The blind pupil, listening, indicates the direction it has taken. The same with heavy objects flung on the ground, a certain distance away. Determine this distance in steps.

14. Sing a series of sounds, while simultaneously attempting to note the rhythms of a stick striking the ground; also other sounds sung by the master in counterpoint.

15. All the exercises for recognising sounds and keys contained in the three volumes of my method entitled: *"Les gammes et les tonalités, le phrasé et les nuances."**

So far I have endeavoured to speak only of the physiological aspect of my attempts, to insist only on the advantages, physical and mental, which, in my opinion, may be afforded by a series of studies immediately aiming at the perfecting of the touch, the development of the

* Jobin et Cie, Lausanne.

sense of space and direction. Before concluding, however, I wish to say something of what a rational study of the elements of sound in music, in their melodic, harmonic, dynamic, rhythmic and agogic combinations can and should exercise upon the imagination and the moral sense of the blind. To initiate them into music with its emotional capabilities and pacificatory influence is also to give ideal form to their most secret aspirations and to make it possible for them to enter into direct communication with normal people.

Of all the arts, music is the one best capable of expressing the instinctive needs of the human being and momentarily fixing in striking and clearly-defined images his aspirations after higher spiritual states. The more thoroughly man enters into possession of his bodily means of expression, the more will the stirrings of his soul assert themselves in transparent beauty and quiet harmony. So many tempestuous desires and unreasoning aspirations assail normal beings like ourselves, as well as the blind, that we are all conscious of an imperious necessity for giving them an elastic and supple form which, while checking their evil influences, will make it possible for desire to vibrate endlessly without compromising the equilibrium of our feelings and sensations. To abandon oneself, body and soul, to music which represents the whole of our powers and determinations, our desires and their realisations, our forward impulses and retrogressions, is to free ourselves from all such perplexities as result from the conflict between our imagination and our vital acts. Music realises the conceptions of our imagination once we have become capable of fathoming the vitality of its artistic functioning. It excites and soothes us at the same time, enables us to divine the future in the present and realise the present in the future. Far from depriving our dreams of any charm they possess, musical education enables us closely to unite the dream with the reality, and the more profoundly a blind man fathoms the secrets of the intimate construction of musical sounds, the more he too will be thrilled by the magic of his evocations. From a strictly utilitarian point of view, a musical education that aims not only at the development of the auditory and musical faculties of the blind man, but also at the development of his muscular sense and his consciousness of time, in all their nuances, is calculated to enable him to collaborate effectively with a sighted person in teaching musical Eurhythmics. A blind musician rightly educated can collaborate with teachers well gifted for Eurhythmics but badly trained from the auditory point of view; so that there will open up before him a new career, alike interesting and useful. And even if this new object here indicated were to be attained only after much groping and hesitation, surely all friends of progress ought to pursue it with the utmost confidence and perseverance. Who knows but that some day it may be the blind man who will inform the normal person as to the possibilities offered by the possession of a complete motor-tactile sense?

I have pointed out a path to be followed, and I sincerely hope that some will be found bold enough to make up their mind to enter it, even at a cost of a certain amount of discomfiture. Assuredly the problem of education is one of those which interest us most passionately in these difficult times. It is worth while giving oneself wholeheartedly to so great an enterprise, with a confident hope in the future, and making every needed sacrifice for the improvement of the race and the mental and moral security of the generations to come.

IX

MUSIC AND SOLIDARITY
(1924)

In beginning a school of music and guiding it along a path of continuous progress, I have always thought that it is not sufficient to bring together a body of eminent professors, to draw up a definite time-table, and to organise interesting concerts. In addition to such things, and more important than all else, is the need to instil into both teachers and taught such an *esprit de corps* and sense of solidarity as will make them of one mind, give unity to their collective experiences, and give them a fresh outlook and a new understanding of things.

The professors ought to have a simultaneous understanding of the various educational methods employed in the school. Those who teach the theory of music should have some knowledge of the means by which the instrumental teachers transform theory into practice, and these latter teachers should, as far as possible, respect the æsthetic laws laid down by the former, so that mutual sacrifice may increase that unity which is indispensable in general musical training. It is also important that the students be invited and encouraged to meet frequently, so that they may learn to know one another, both as human beings and as artists. There must be established between them such relations as are based on mutual esteem and sympathy, on a laudable instinct of emulation that never degenerates into the mean and paltry rivalry that has been known to distinguish certain types of competitive examinations.

There is nothing better calculated to develop this spirit of combination than debates among the pupils themselves, with teachers or professors in the chair, in the course of which general questions dealing with æsthetics or philosophy are discussed. The professors should also have periodical meetings (to which the students would not be admitted), in order to exchange their impressions of the students, and so supplement and complete the opinions they have already formed regarding the ability, temperament, and character of their pupils. Indeed, it is often extremely difficult to form a clear and adequate judgment of a pupil whom one is training in only one of the several branches of music. Music is an art as many-sided as life itself; it is impossible to fathom all its secrets; and only by encountering obstacles and difficulties of various kinds may it be explored. How frequently does it happen, for instance, that a teacher of the pianoforte accuses some pupil of lack of musical ability solely because muscular or nervous antagonisms make it impossible for the player to summon those resources of expression that are nevertheless latent within him: for to express badly what one feels is not the same thing as having no feelings to express. What is important is first to develop the sensibility of the pupil, then to discover the best way of directing his nervous activities along the right channel, and to stimulate an intimate association between a pupil's impressions and his mode of expression.

Again, how frequently it happens that the theoretical master bewails the poor quality of the work of certain students who, though naturally and instinctively musical and capable of the highest flights of imagination, are repelled by the mathematical aspect of their harmony exercises. Such a feeling frequently arises from a lack of power of concentration. The whole of the specialised studies should come under the same system of analysis, comparison and deduction. All fixed lines of demarcation between instruction in aural training, harmony, rhythmics, composition, and musical history, should be abolished. It is essential that each student be compelled to form part of a choral or instrumental ensemble, and inevitably be induced to take an interest in the studies as a whole. The various modes of instruction should all work together. It is only by living in an atmosphere completely permeated with art, during the course of their musical studies, that students will feel growing and developing in them that clear judgment and ardent love without which the future artist will always remain incomplete as a human being.

To the love and knowledge of art, the curiosity aroused by the analysis of musical compositions, and the joy created by sensations of sound and by spiritual and emotional communion with great works, should be added sympathy with the efforts of others, respect for fellow-individuals, and an earnest desire to unite with them to make common progress. This instinct of solidarity should be awakened in early youth, and it is for schools of music to develop and advance this instinct by every possible means even, if necessary, at the sacrifice of certain secondary branches of the curriculum. Indeed, their role consists not only in training future musicians in their art, but also in developing their sense of *esprit de corps*, in teaching them not only to create and interpret, but also to live.

X

UNITY IN MUSICAL EDUCATION
(1922)

THE education of the people is in process of becoming more socialised. The chief tendency of present-day teaching is to subordinate the education of individuals to that of a well-organised mass, then to elicit the emergence of special personalities from their environment, and lastly to set up relations between individuals and groups. It is surely time – since educational concerns are manifestly as poignant as economic considerations – to think of setting up relations between the various schools and academies of music in which our children learn to sing, to listen, to interpret and to judge music.

It is quite evident that the question of competition plays no part whatsoever in this dispersal of educational resources. Each institution has its own clientele, and there is no desire on the part of teachers to capture pupils, to the detriment of rival schools. Each school, however, pursues a personal object, seeks to set up special musical surroundings, to contrast its own tendencies with those of the rest, and to create a particular environment. This method is certainly justifiable, since in artistic matters teaching is of value only in so far as the teacher possesses those qualities of authority, originality, and all-round knowledge which are capable of making instruction a permanent acquisition.

Nevertheless, art assumes various forms; the artistic temperament shows itself in many ways, and the would-be musician needs to study in more than one school if he is to unfold his own distinctive personality. Is it not clear that those who control the musical movement should keep to one general idea, imparting to one another and mutually benefiting by their ideas and experiences? If we set up our own powers against other powers, do we not thereby lessen and weaken them? But if we pool our wills and capacities, outline a common programme of study which each can follow out in his own particular way, are we not thereby drawing nearer the goal of all musical study: to enable the people to love and understand the great masterpieces? And would not such a result fill every teacher with that indefinable, that exalted joy afforded by community of ideas and the attempt to bring people together? Indeed, the harmonising of musical temperaments ought to be identical with that of sounds: dissonances, yes; but also a plan in composition, the subordination of harmonies to a leading melody freely pursued, and the sacrifice of individual interests to a general idea. . . .

Universities are everywhere, to some extent, attempting to exchange professors, to create a world-wide scientific movement, to provoke exchange of ideas. The recent initiative taken by many members of universities in all countries is calculated to make national temperaments more pliant and flexible, to increase the powers of imagination, to make intellectual and vital reactions more keen and spontaneous, to circulate streams of more intense life among antagonistic minds. It seems to me — at a time in history when Switzerland, from the intellectual, social and political point of view, appears to have become a sort of central laboratory in which the most incongruous ideas clash and interpenetrate, and then amalgamate under the influence of a common desire for mutual understanding — that the principal *conservatoires* of each country might endeavour to enter into direct relations with one another, organise meetings at the beginning of each season, at which the delegates of different schools would expound their ideas, and seek to establish a common programme of study, so as to set up examinations of equal value, analogous to those in vogue between the various universities.

Neither officially nor semi-officially is there any relation whatsoever between the different musical schools of each country. Why is this? Is it really necessary that all musical instruction should be so specialised that a student, on leaving the musical schools of London, Paris, or Rome, for instance, should not be able to continue at the *conservatoires* of Geneva or Zurich, without sitting for a fresh examination and, as is frequently the case, taking up his studies again from the beginning?

It would be easy to devise a general programme of musical studies, comprising, in the case of the French *conservatoires*, instruction based more especially on an acquaintance with the works and methods of Latin composers, and in the case of British schools of music, on a knowledge of the works of Anglo-Saxon writers. This must, of course, be regarded from the standpoint of temperament rather than from that of science, for manifestly no one school of music can restrict itself to the study of the musical productions of a single race. But, after all, it cannot be denied that the study of the methods and processes of Debussy, Ravel, and other modern representatives of the French school – as also that of the methods of composers allied to the Latin school, such as Moussorgsky, Stravinsky, etc. – could not be as systematically pursued in London, Zurich, or New York, as it could be in Paris. On the other hand, French music teachers less frequently offer examples of style from the works of Mahler, Strauss, Reger, Brahms, and Schönberg than is the case in German Switzerland or America. It is unnecessary to speak of such pioneers as Rameau, Couperin, Froberger or Buxtehude, whose composition models are very differently interpreted, according to the *conservatoire* at which our young people study.

And yet . . . human emotions are the same in every country. Styles, modes and forms may be different; but impulses are identical. A musician can only go through a complete course of study if he is acquainted with the styles and temperaments of the two great schools whose rhythms are creating a universal musical current. Hence, would it not be well from time to time to effect an exchange of teachers between the conservatoires of various countries, or even between the principal music schools of the same country? Nowadays travelling is more difficult and expensive than before the war: it is important that musical education should not have to suffer on that account.

Music is a world language, one that cannot be understood unless we have been initiated into its many and diverse forms by means of teaching that is both flexible and adaptable. If the principal *conservatoires* would but agree to exchange certain classes in style, their pupils, on leaving, would have a solid and extensive knowledge of their subject, and would not be compelled to travel afterwards in order to imbibe the artistic conceptions of the musicians of other races.

Music neither should nor can be nationalised. The history of musical development proves to us the constant influence of the temperament of one people over the rest, of a single genius over several races. Such an exchange of teachers and professors as is here advocated would prove beneficial not only to individuals but to society as a whole.

XI

THE MUSICAL EDUCATION OF THE FUTURE

(1922)

DURING a recent visit to England I have been greatly interested and filled with a daily increasing admiration at seeing the attempts that are being made in that land by a considerable number of artists and teachers to ensure for the young people new facilities of education and more favourable conditions of existence. Almost everywhere in the United Kingdom tentative efforts show a tendency to infuse a more human character into school studies, to call forth in the child greater freedom of action and thought, and, by educating both will and imagination, to prepare the ground for a more complete expansion of physical and mental powers. The interesting work carried on at Geneva by the Institut Jean-Jacques Rousseau has its analogue in England, and if Spencer, pioneer and emancipator, were to return to earth, he would have just occasion to be proud of his followers. From the educational point of view, England has become a land of liberty; there all kinds of projects and schemes for scholastic reform are welcomed with greater interest than is the case in Latin countries, where, as Montaigne expresses it, "the laws of consciousness are born, not of nature, but of custom, each individual having the utmost veneration for the manners and opinions approved of and recognised by those around him, neither detaching himself from them without remorse, nor adopting them without approbation."

From the strictly musical standpoint English private schools have made remarkable progress. Old educational traditions are no longer kept up except in certain large official establishments. Everywhere else recourse is had to new methods, the object of which is mainly to develop the musical sense of the pupils and to familiarise them with variations both in substance and in form before special study is made of any particular instrument, or a headlong plunge into effects of virtuosity is attempted.

Owing to the kindness of the general inspector of musical education, we attended, in various London schools, "music" lessons which were really deserving of the name, lessons in which imitation exercises play but a secondary part, where the hearing faculties are developed with particular care, and attempts at improvisation precede pianoforte study strictly so called. For instance, it was our privilege to hear all the pupils in a class of children from twelve to fifteen – unprepared for our visit – improvise, as they sang and accompanied themselves on the pianoforte, little songs perfect as regards form, adapted to themes which we had set them. In this new kind of education, the analysis of the classic forms – minuet, rondo, gavotte, etc. – occupies a prominent role, and this department of study is begun in the very first year of instruction, whereas in our case it is scarcely ever undertaken except at the end of the course, a most unreasonable method to adopt. An executive interpretation of pianoforte works of various forms, without the possibility of understanding the mind which produced these forms, gives the pupil nothing but a very superficial knowledge of his subject.

As Joubert says: 'Thoughts must spring from the soul, words from thoughts, and sentences from words.' Education should enable us to give form in our thought, and any form that is dictated only by memory and not by temperament is of an inferior type. To enable the budding musician to recognise if the musical phrase played on the pianoforte is by Bach, by Handel, by Haydn, or by Mozart, after he has been shown the differences in temperament and mode of expression which characterise these masters, is an exercise in which at the end of each lesson, all the pupils in the classes we visited take great delight. It was a real joy to note with what animation the children worked and to what an extent their musical taste and analytical sense were already developed.

Mention has just been made of powers of imitation. These, instead of being cultivated for the sole purpose of enabling the pupil to reproduce the time and tone-shades dictated by the teacher, are, in the new schools here mentioned, directly utilised in studies of harmony and form. The teacher plays a short passage which the pupil endeavours to reproduce from memory on a second pianoforte. This method, vaguely suggested by Mathis Lussy, and employed by ourselves for over a score of years, is far more capable of making a child musical than are the current systems which develop the faculties of sight and touch rather than those of hearing, indispensable though these latter are to the musician. Studies in improvisation, when based on the consciousness of a correct balancing of phrases, as well as on that of natural harmonic connections, quite naturally prepare the pupil for the understanding and analysis of musical works and enable him to regard and sense music as a true language, a natural means of expression.

It is related that Anatole France, who had been requested to say which was the best of French grammars, declared that frequent oral improvisation, under the supervision of a master who insists on balance of periods and exactness of terms, constitutes a means of instruction far superior to the logical study of the most ingenious grammar book in the world. It is the same with music. However, we must of course not confuse the exercises in improvisation here recommended – rapid composition in obedience to the laws of form, rhythm, and harmony – with the structureless ramblings, devoid both of plan and of development, by which so many *backfisch* both male and female, old and young, complaisantly attempt to interpret their muddled thinking. All education, whether physical, moral, artistic, religious, or political, should be built up on respect for order and proportion, balance and style. No mere theoretical instruction can bring about the development in youthful musicians of the desire for beauty, the consciousness of self, the will to act, the power to construct. It is more important to give future artists a general trend of mind than to elicit progress in them by various accumulated means of expression devoid alike of order and of connection, or by experiments that are not based on the interaction of sensation and feeling. To quicken the mind is good, but to quicken the temperament in order to place it under the control of the mind is even better. That the curriculum should be varied and the professors and teachers numerous, gifted and renowned, is not enough. In a school of music, as in any other school, there must be the ever-present desire to create in the pupils an inner moral and artistic life together with the will and determination to develop not only their musical faculties but also those qualities of judgment and discipline, of integrity and solidarity, of initiative and perseverance, without which the most richly endowed and well-trained musician will never be other than a poor, worthless individual, incapable either of steering his own course through life or of contributing towards the development of the race.

ART

XII

EURHYTHMICS AND ART

(1925)

THE sensations afforded by the natural rhythms of our bodies strengthen our instinct for rhythm and create rhythmic consciousness. It is through this instinct and this consciousness, blended with the æsthetic sense, that we experience complete artistic emotions. For an artist, emotion is not only the outcome of nervous, physical and instinctive vibrations; it should spring from that mysterious laboratory where physical sensations become transformed by higher energies and wills. Undoubtedly, the artist is generally born such, one whose organism often functions apart from consciousness. The manifestations of subconsciousness, however, are not adequate to create works of art, for art cannot dispense with order and harmony, and these two factors depend on the conscious ego.

The consciousness of rhythm is the power to grasp the relations between physical and intellectual movements and to experience the modifications caused in these movements by the impulses of emotion and thought. By way of the concept created by movement, the artist should return to the cause of the motor sensations experienced and to the original generating emotion. The keenly sensitive listener or spectator should on his side recapture sensation by way of emotion, and rediscover the creative thought. True æsthetic emotion is felt only when emotion and sensation are blended in unity of concept. As

Edouard Schuré says: "Idea is the generating-point of beauty. Idea produces the form which shapes matter, as spirit creates the soul which weaves the body."

In beginning to study the laws and effects of rhythm, mind works upon matter. But any complete education should endeavour to raise matter to the plane of mind, otherwise it is ineffectual. To make an instrument is insufficient; this instrument must be placed at the service of thought. The purely gymnastic element in our lessons aims at the development of health and physical harmony; the study of the relations between movements tends to develop order in the body. But shall we rest content with gaining health, harmony, and order? No, the result is inadequate unless we effect a synthesis. From the harmonious co-operation of strength and suppleness, of beauty of attitude and of rhythm, art and emotion must be born.

Originally rhythm of sounds and rhythm of movements formed one unity, but they have become separate in the course of time. This special education should lead us to rediscover rhythm at its source, to acquire fuller æsthetic consciousness. The development of energy and activity inspires in us an increasing need of æsthetic pleasure and favours the acquisition of new faculties as well as the resurrection of original ones. It is a new art that we are, quite naturally, invited to construct, new to our times, because its conception has long been distorted by a love of æsthetic complications and its elementary form degraded by ornamental additions – because it proceeds solely from our essential vital functions and from our purest energies, whence spring all our concepts of beauty.

A few lessons in rhythmic gymnastics suffice to show that ugliness of movement dwells in the movement itself, not in ugliness of body. If the movement betrays artifice, and if effort is apparent, the result is ugly. Most æsthetes agree that grace of movement results from the ease born of mechanical perfection. Doubtless they are right. Daily practice obviously brings about the elimination of such elements as are unnecessary for action, as well as the reduction of effort to a minimum. If the suppleness of certain movements is devoid of effeminacy, the ease with which they are performed gives the impression of grace — but ease is not always harmony, which should emanate from the entire personality. The slightest trace of a desire to appear graceful destroys the total effect. Does an impression of bodily grace imply a perfect impression of beauty? Not always, for perfect beauty of movement cannot dispense with rhythm. Now, a graceful movement which seems to us beautiful, repeated again and again in time though without rhythm, inevitably produces an impression of monotony. There is no beauty that does not evoke an idea of the renewal and continuation of life.

Examine certain traditional figures of the classic Italian ballet. Could anything be less moving than the spectacle of fifty *danseuses* obstinately bent upon inclining the head in one direction and raising the leg in the other? If a succession of movements is to be beautiful, the duration and intensity of the rhythms must vary, the imagination must come into play in order to create contrasts and alternations. We should feel the presence of a guiding mind which, profiting by momentary impulses, prevents movements from becoming automatic. The introduction of spontaneous rhythmic movements into a succession of ordered movements inevitably calls forth emotion. But even without this intervention of natural impulses, a series of conscious movements subjected to a varied succession of rhythms will give an impression of beauty and harmony. If choreography is to be revivified, it needs to acquire new motor habits, brought into being both by instinct and by consciousness. Its technique need not be changed, but it should be supplemented by a knowledge of bodily nuances in relation to those of time. This new study will enable us to define the laws which govern the mutual relations between the rhythm of sounds and that of movements.*

Even the best of the modern ballets – and there are some very fine ones – give the impression that the dancers interpret the music in wholly external fashion, while on the other hand the composers of tonal rhythms, intended for expression by the human body, are ignorant of the laws of bodily movement. Neither dancer nor composer understands that the ballet is a complex of two arts, the plastic and the musical, which ought to combine and contrast with each other, to act together and also separately. These two arts have been so long dissociated that the public has forgotten that they were originally one. During a performance of the ballet how many musicians see nothing, how many plastic artists have their ears stopped! Isadora Duncan, to whom the art of dancing is indebted for a healthy return to simplicity and emotion, attempted to revive the Greek art of moving plastic. She did not, however, appear to be sufficiently aware, as were the Greeks, that the rhythm of dancing is closely connected with the movements of sound, with the rhythms of music and language. It is through these latter that reality emerges out of appearance.

From the union of language and music – song, lyrical drama – will never be born anything but a secondary art if the poetry of the words is transformed into sound poetry of a different style, if musical rhythms do not constantly agree with verbal rhythms in their oppositions and con-

* See "The Cinema and its Music," p. 202 *et seq.*

trasts as in their blendings, and if each of these means of
expression does not consent to certain necessary sacrifices.* Similarly the art of dancing, if it still insists on
union with music, should achieve the transmutation of
sound into bodily movement and of movement into sound.
It is not enough that moving plastic should be super-
imposed on music. It should spring forth from music as a
spontaneous growth, adapt music's external form and
style to its own, and interpret all its shades of emotion.
Such transposition is possible only through a dual education, which is needed by even the most gifted and talented
artists.

Watch the Russian dancers, whose technique is perfect, their gracefulness natural and simple, and their
temperament of unrivalled expressiveness; see them
attempt the bodily interpretation of the tranquil and
sustained element in music, to rhythms with a continuous
tranquil flow, with no jolts or emotional shocks. Are not
their innate powers of spontaneous expression occasionally inadequate to the bodily expression of gradations in
time and energy — the *mezzopiano* and *rubato* of tonal
phrases? Their wonderful leaps and voltes, their impetuous gestures, their fantastic evolutions amid dazzling
stage effects and flashing lights — all this gives extraordinary brilliance to their interpretations. But just as,
in order not to spoil the effects of the painted scenery,
their illumination is frequently compelled to dispense with
the art of nuance, so — for lack of having studied the
relations between the different *tempi*, from *allegro* to
larghetto, and those which rhythm sets up between the
different degrees of energy — the Russians as a rule only
interpret perfectly the violent or fantastic passages of the
music they have to express, and not the parts that indicate
restrained tenderness and poignant intimacy. Perfect art

* See "The Cinema and its Music," p. 199.

will not be seen on the stage until musicians are better acquainted with the resources of the human body, and until dancers learn the natural laws of musical rhythm.*

The fusion of the two fundamental elements of music was respected by the Greeks. The idea was expressed rhythmically by sounds or by words, the plastic form was achieved synchronically, harmonically and rhythmically, by bodily movements. The love of the Greeks for clarity, for health and beauty, impelled them to give first place to the plastic element in musical expression, but musical unity nevertheless was not thereby impaired.

Moreover, dancing – to us an æsthetic pastime – appeared to the Greeks as an act of faith, including art and philosophy. Later on, Christianity broke the unity between matter and spirit, teaching men to despise the body and to seek after the Beautiful solely in the abstract. The result was that in music the mystical element was more specially cultivated, and rhythm had to find refuge in the architecture of cathedrals. Music forgot its origin, which is in the dance, and men lost, not only in art but in everyday life, the instinct for expressive and harmonious movements. Their mental faculties became hyper-trophied in proportion as their sense instincts were re-pressed. Heredity intensified these exaggerations, and even created emotions which the body had never before experienced. Is it not important for the child's happiness in his early development that education should reveal to him, above all else, those elementary feelings which have their root in his true nature? Rhythmic gymnastics acts equally upon the subconscious and the conscious.

Concerning the participation of the unconscious in the creation of art, it has been said that, if in everyone there

* See "The Technique of Moving Plastic," p. 44; also "The Inner Technique of Rhythm," p. 60.

dwells a being almost unknown to us, who whispers words and thoughts and inspires us to do things frequently opposed to the temperament we imagine to be ours – then the origin of this subconscious assistance is none the less in our conscious personality or in that of our ancestors. It is well known that many people write better than they speak and are unable to express themselves truly except on paper. This might be regarded as an intervention of the subconscious, though as a matter of fact it is simply association of ideas. When we concentrate on a given subject, there is set up a whole series of vibrations which rouses the entire mechanism of our ideas and feelings. Innumerable associations form, blending with one another. Their effect is so unexpected that we forget the initial sensations which called them forth. The manifestations of the subconscious appear not to obey logic, though frequently they are but the unforeseen consequence of forgotten impulses. It is rare that the ground of our consciousness is prepared to give way before the unexpected putting-forth of secret forces seeking to issue from the depths of our sensible nature.

And so, since our entire spiritual life originates in the co-operation between our conscious and our unconscious nature, the educator has a dual part to play. He should endeavour, on the one hand, to put the child in possession of all his conscious powers of expression; and, on the other hand, to enable him to recover lost instincts and to summon forth in him the greatest possible number of instinctive manifestations of every kind. He must develop the conscious "self" of the child so as to enable him to see the danger of certain bad habits and to struggle effectively against them. He must also enquire which, of all the subconscious manifestations he awakens, may be cultivated by the conscious mind. Newton, when asked how he succeeded in discovering the law of gravitation, replied: "By continually thinking about it!" There always comes a moment when continuous and conscious effort finally elicits the revelation of the subconscious idea. "There is such a thing," wrote Schopenhauer, "as an 'unconscious rumination of thought.'" Nevertheless, there are people who do not perform this action naturally: they have to be taught to ruminate! Thought should not wait passively for the aid of the subconscious revelation, it should summon it with all its might and be constantly prepared for an unexpected visit. But while it is necessary that education should enable us to analyse the various forms of emotion, it should not incite us to analyse the principle of our emotion itself. Eurhythmics should awaken simple perceptions which, along the lines of association, lead to a fuller emotional development. This is the natural interpretation of the emotion which constitutes art. Both body and mind may be trained to achieve this interpretation in accordance with the laws of rhythm.

There are, of course, emotions of a non-physical origin. "Mystical emotion is an intensification of æsthetic emotion and proceeds from a state of mind akin to intoxication. Consequently, it is followed by a reaction." All emotions susceptible of bodily expression are not necessarily sensorial, but the bodily expression invites a style which makes them æsthetic. It is often said that art should imitate nature; it would be more correct to say that art should be inspired by – and embellish – nature.

Often nature is but partially beautiful. Similarly, some emotions contain only certain elements of beauty. It is the function of art to select from among these elements. To express an emotion plastically, the form adopted must be beautiful, but must not conceal the emotion, for expression of this latter would then become incomprehensible. The Greeks sacrificed emotion to harmony of form. The Christians of an entire epoch sacrificed form to the expression of such feelings as grief, repentance, and death. Those who, by a special form of education, wish to help their fellow-beings to rehabilitate the cult of moving beauty, ought to take care not to deprive æsthetic emotion of hereditary instinctive elements. It is not enough to take, just as they are, the emotions resulting from the contingencies of life and nature. To create a work of art we need a superior intellect. This intellect is the product of the equilibrium and the harmony we should try to introduce into our movements and therefore into our minds. The way to attain this end is to study the laws of rhythm, which include the laws of art, and which, once we have mastered them, will be the means of embellishing and ennobling our everyday life.

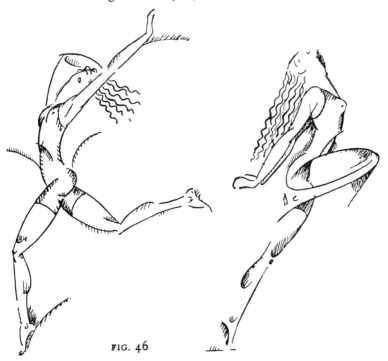

FIG. 46

XIII

THE CINEMA AND ITS MUSIC *
(1925)

THE progress made by the cinema has been so rapid that there is nothing to be wondered at if its admirers, in the course of the past twenty years, have been compelled to modify their opinions, frequently, and to their own amazement. As regards myself, fifteen years ago I had occasion to write an article on the relations existing between music and the cinema: three years ago I wrote another, in which I repudiated with the utmost conviction the opinions expressed in the first. Now, on chancing to read the English translation of my recent article which I regarded as definitive and ultimate, I am astonished to discover a fresh modification – this time brought about in a very short space of time – of the ideas I held as to the expediency of sound music blended with image music, and the variations imposed upon musical style by the changing nature of moving visions.

Some time ago I had the joy of seeing the first films of the Lumière brothers on the Boulevard des Italiens. They were a striking revelation to me. There was no musical accompaniment, and I distinctly remember that I did not regret a silence which I even thought impressive. The visual effects of these films were of an essentially dynamic and rhythmic character. The rise and fall of the waves needed no accompaniment, for they themselves created musical emotions of the most extraordinary inten-

* Although the "talkies" have recently evinced a considerable improvement on the music composed for cinematograph performances, it may be of interest to the reader to reprint here the present article originally issued in 1925. The reader will notice that most of the improvements of the last two years correspond with the desiderata expressed in this article, at a time when the music of the cinema performed nothing but the mere function of accompaniment.

192

sity. The "train entering the station" seemed graduated
after the traditional laws of tonal *rallentando*. Assuredly,
the aid of music seemed quite unnecessary for a spectacle
presented with such natural rhythm and nuance.

Doubtless pianoforte accompaniment was introduced
because the films covered a wide field and occupied the
spectator for a whole evening. . . . The public, seated
in utter darkness and in absolute silence, had no opportunity, as in a theatre, of stretching their legs at intervals.
Besides, music, probably unaware of its power, did not
at first participate artistically in the spectacle. Doubtless
a skilful pianist attempted to avoid too flagrant a contrast
of style between the music and the moving picture. He
shrewdly played valses and polkas, nocturnes and tangos,
quick-step pieces and Chopin's 'Funeral March,' and this
sufficed to please the *élite* of the public. Then came a day
when some sensitive and far-seeing pianist noticed the
peculiar intensity of certain emotional gestures when they
happened to coincide with accentuations of sound. After
that, he contrived to find additional opportunities of making the dynamics of sight coincide with those of music.
This attempt to obtain concurrence of energy was admired
and generally imitated, for there is no intelligent invention which is not immediately plagiarised when it is dis-
covered to have an undoubted effect upon snobs and
simple-minded people. Then a composer had an idea of
improvising special music which followed as exactly as
possible the style and rhythm of the action and aimed at
interpreting the various shades of emotion. This inno-
vation was very successful with spectators particularly
sensitive to musical rhythm and who – probably with no
definite idea of the new role played by the art of sound –
observed on the screen an increase of life and in their own
bodies a special animation which brought them into more
direct communication with the spectacle.

Meanwhile, the style of cinematographic production was gradually modified. The films increased in length, while their characteristic rhythms became shorter and alternated more frequently with divers secondary rhythms which created a host of contrasts. The *leit-motif* was introduced, breaking into the regular periods or creating short polyrhythms. It became difficult for the improviser to keep to a continuous and regular style of playing. The ever-increasing gradations of action and the dispersion of images into picturesque accessory illustrations detracted from the unity of style and from the organisation of the musical accompaniment. Whereas a certain number of extemporisers insisted on details of images, those of a more artistic type, *i.e.* more respectful of the laws that govern the continuous developments of the musical idea, tried to eliminate from their playing all superfluous graces and occasional picturesque effects, and, instead, to devise "continuous" music, indifferent to minor details and bent solely upon creating an enveloping atmosphere for the development of the action depicted – a sort of stage effect in sound.

Other pianists, orchestras also, were content to choose, from classic or modern composers, such music as approximately expressed the general character of the various dramatic episodes; composers also, with the same object and following like tendencies, wrote symphonic works intended to illustrate a film from beginning to end.

On their side, the producers of films, influenced by the sound vibrations all round, became aware of the musical nature of their work and tried to portray a sort of visual music, terminologically copied from the other, *i.e.* having melodies and harmonies, counterpoints, developments, and orchestration. A fresh attempt to find rhythms based on fluctuations of light and shade, alternations of straight, curved and broken lines, of measured or spontaneous movements, and of pauses dictated by the need of rest or the intervention of emotional breaks — gave their productions a more original aspect. They tried to produce on the screen veritable symphonies which, comprising as they did thematic developments, seemed to them to correspond to musical symphonies. . . . All that henceforth was necessary — they said to themselves — was to superimpose one symphony upon the other, and so blend the various plastic and sound elements, the shifting figure and the melody, the evolutions and the counterpoint, the combinations of individual or collective gestures and the harmony. Thus they imagined they were creating a new artistic association wherein would blend space and time, linear construction and lyric form, light vibrations and sound vibrations, bodily rhythms and musical rhythms. To do this, however, they did not dream of submitting to the intimate experiences necessary to produce musical sensibility. They were ignorant alike of the metaphysical essence of music and of the technical means of imparting to music physical faculties of expression. Musicians were equally ignorant of that particular technique without which all collaboration becomes an illusion. As Appia well says:

"If music would control the mobility of the body, it must first find out what the body expects from it, then it will consider this and try to develop within itself the faculty required, a faculty that will depend strictly on what is offered in return. Music can give nothing vital to the body unless it first receives life from the body. This is evident. And so the body gives up its own life to music, to receive it back again, though now organised and transfigured." *

To make vital the collaboration they desire, producers should deliberately abjure the magical lure of words and phrases, repudiate all idealogical speculation, and examine alike "the soul and the body" of two arts quite distinct,

* Adolphe Appia, "L'Œuvre d'art vivant" (Edition Atar, Paris, 26 rue St. Dominique). See "The Inner Technique of Rhythm," p. 60.

though equal in expressive value. The first appeals directly to the eye and would exercise this privilege constantly, whereas the second, aware that it is entrusted with but a second-rate role, accepts the situation and aims only at strengthening visual impressions. Before blending two elements, is it not necessary to study thoroughly their nature, their peculiarities and their powers?

First of all, in the musical accompaniment of the films, there are technical means of expression which have become traditional. Although their effects are wholly external and are already largely out of date, it is advisable to mention them here, for after all they result from a natural observation of visual and tonal equivalences. The style of an epoch (costumes, architecture, general aspect of the characters) is musically transposed very easily by the use of melodic and harmonic rules dictated, along the ages, by the environment, social conditions and particular circumstances of individual life. . . . The natural stage-scenery (mountains, lakes, meadows, forests) may be musically expressed by certain sequences of chords, by the special nature of rhythms and keys. . . . The general pace of the action, slow or swiftly moving, continuous or broken, clearly corresponds to the various *tempi*, (*andante, allegro, presto con fuoco, allegretto grazioso, esitando, calmato*, etc.) of the music. Gradations of light and shade correspond to those of intensity and timbre. Space itself may, to some extent, be represented by musical harmonies that are open or close, complete or imperfect. For instance, a succession of chords deprived of their thirds inevitably gives an impression of peace, of continuity and boundless horizons, making them suggestive of quiet meadows, vast stretches of ocean, a virgin snowfield, or the quiet shadows of a cathedral.

The prominent feature of a character may be rendered by major, minor and chromatic keys, and the interplay

of these keys. . . . The several manifestations of temperament need special rhythms, all of which may be trans-
muted into sound-rhythms, by means of concordant
dynamic forces or synchronous accentuations. . . . Continuous gestures may be represented by a flow of smooth
continuous sounds, sudden gestures by *staccato*, hesitation
by syncopation. Sequences of gestures, attitudes and
changes of place constituting a whole are readily transposed into musical phrases and periods; their several
degrees of intensity and fullness are naturally rendered
by the many shades of tonal intensity, by *ff*, *pp*, *crescendo*
and *decrescendo*. Finally, the cessation of human movement and the fall of light may be rightly expressed by the
rest in music. . . . Obviously such transpositions as these
are quite elementary and artificial, relating solely to
technical knowledge which has only an apparent affinity
with art itself. To be an artist is to possess the dual faculty,
first of thinking, then of "expanding one's thought into
life." Once certain spiritualised sensations are converted
into powerful images, the artist will always find means of
giving them expressive form. "The artist," says Peladan,
"is the man who has consciously set up a concordat
between his psychic personality and universal science, in
balanced accord with life and the ideal."

Certainly then there are many ways of blending aural
and visual impressions. In a musico-plastic alliance, however, it is important that each of the allied arts should
express itself in its personal form, while respecting, at
the cost of certain sacrifices, the natural form of the other.
This form is subordinated to the nature of the organs that
have to perceive and register sensations. And so, down
the ages there have been set up certain types of tonal
architecture which time can modify but not distort. The
laws of musical phrasing are immutable, those of melodic
development vary only as regards their length, *i.e.* the

frequency of their identical or varied repetitions. The forms of the visual symphony have not yet been determined. The seventh art is hesitant among a number of new possibilities; it is so young and vital that it is continually being carried off into hitherto unexplored fields; assured of success, it is quite ready to throw away the forms it momentarily adopts as soon as it glimpses the possibility of conceiving new ones. How could it accept any definite ultimate style when it constantly sees its means of expression grow in number?

It desires an alliance with musical art, but does not feel the need of abandoning, even temporarily, its attempts to acquire a style of its own in order to conform to the traditions of an allied art which it regards at bottom as subordinate – and probably with good reason. Music is well aware that it is for her to modify herself in order to espouse the cause of an entirely new art which is affirmed to be her brother, but which, for the time being, she recognises only as an adopted brother. The projected and mutually consenting union has not yet come about: it will take place only on quite special conditions – the same as those which secured the partnership existing between words and music.

In the song, poetry and music make mutual concessions. Each possesses stereotyped forms, created by incessant experiments, and yet we find now the one, now the other, of these arts refusing to assert itself in order to obey those laws of alternation and contrast which ensure the happy equilibrium of the elements to be harmonised. Music does not follow the words of a poem; it endeavours to draw out their essence. With its own means of expression it reproduces the productive emotion of the poem, completes the action of the word, expands and widens its province. Although it takes account of the rhythms of speech, music does not on that account relinquish its own particular rhythms but fashions them so as to blend more intimately with the thought that created the verbal rhythms. The reason is that it feels the impossibility of collaborating with poetry except by respecting its original forms, both internal and external. . . . The poem continually accepts modifications imposed by alliance with music which breaks it up and annotates it. And when it comes to an end, after expressing itself fully, it leaves its ally complete liberty to extend the generating emotion. It also allows music to modify its time-length, prolonging by three or four times the sounds of the words, developing a musical phrase of two bars during the emission of a single syllable, and so abating its general pace, as well as the particular pace of each part.*

A similar mutual consent will bring about the union of the cinematographic art and the musical art, once the former has made the experiments necessary for self-assertion in a certain number of determinate forms, in movements ordered and regulated by the universal laws of equilibrium. Then two forms will blend, two thoughts will harmonise, whereas, in the present state of things, music that desires close alliance with the moving image finds itself continually thwarted by the accumulation on the screen of effects of extreme variety and interest, but which it cannot attempt to interpret without prejudicing its own personal existence. In the alliance between words and music, we have seen that the musical development inevitably prolongs the time-lengths of the words and phrases, but this in no way injures the continuity of thought, whereas the extraordinary brevity of visual rhythms – the art of the cinema is one of detail – forces the composer who has undertaken to interpret them to abandon all progressive logic, whether æsthetic or sentimental. When we see on the screen all the bells in the

* See "Eurhythmics and Art," p. 187.

steeple pealing forth, it is never for more than fifteen or twenty seconds. It would be childish to expect the music to play this peal of bells, even if, as in one film, the ringing acts as *leit-motif* and is of the utmost importance in the action. Development is necessary for every musical idea, to unite with which the ever-advancing pictorial ideas should also be developed continuously, adapting themselves to definite forms. These forms are probably to be found in slight variations of nuances and progressive modifications of light and movement, during the somewhat prolonged exposure of a typical picture. This latter retains its essential aspect during the music, without the risk of appearing monotonous, since its variations are solely of ornamental and tonal importance.*

Until the cinema re-establishes a style, or series of styles, that can readily be analysed, and acquaintance with which would secure for the musician new possibilities of harmonious collaboration, the present-day film and its complement in sound might at once mutually consent to certain sacrifices to consolidate their union. For instance, the scenic action ought from time to time to relinquish the perpetual movement which too often characterises it, and allow the scenery time to assert its æsthetic or emotional role. Then the music would again come into its own and would comment on the scenery with its own distinctive methods of expression, emphasising its poetical nature, or perhaps evoking the presence of the human beings intended to blend their life with its own.

On the other hand, the music might be vaguely suggested, or even might cease altogether, at times when the action asserts itself fully and categorically, from the rhythmic and dynamic point of view. Indeed, the suggestive and

* In a new film, "Le Dernier des Hommes," without sub-titles, these scenes are developed in a sustained style which is singularly adapted to musical comment.

inciting power of music finally becomes weakened if continuously exercised. In certain cases silence constitutes a quite special state of expressive emotion; in others, it strengthens the capacity for interpreting rhythmic bodily movements. . . . Similarly, the retaining on the screen for a few seconds of the human body and groups of individuals in harmonious attitudes so as to create what are still generally called *tableaux vivants* – would supply the moving plastic art with opportunities for pleasing contrasts. Such arrests of movement would enable the music to convert its lively rhythm into peaceful harmonies, or even to express the inner rhythms of the various characters.

Thus it would be to the advantage of producers to moderate the excesses of the soloists or groups so as not to be continually giving inordinate expression to certain impulsive desires of the characters. These would lose no whit of their emotional power by temporarily diminishing the intensity of their action so as to enable the music to express for them the feelings which so riotously excite them. Moreover, there are certain emotions that are not inevitably represented by grimaces, frowns, gnashing of teeth, chewing of cigars, clenched fists, shaking knees, and glycerine tears! Since the music is there, ever ready to play its expressive role, would it not be preferable to appeal to it occasionally in order to husband the powers of the actors and to avoid giving the impression of artificial disturbance, the disorderly effects of which finally injure and destroy one another and act exclusively on the nervous system, not on the intelligent and nicely graded sensibilities of the spectators?

I am just now thinking of certain unpleasant and disorderly scenes in the Swedish film "Goesta Berling," so lacking in style and unity of proportion that in order to comment on them the music would have to indulge in most utterly extravagant effects. (Fortunately, other Swedish films give impressions of peaceful and harmonious beauty.) The finest disorder – it has been said – is an effect of art; indeed, certain forms of disorder, born of the clash of blind forces, may produce on the masses an irresistible dynamic effect, without making any artistic impression. But an impression of harmony may also emerge from scenes of fevered agitation, if this agitation has been made rhythmic. The most stirring human conflicts can be quite distinctively filmed without losing anything of their rugged vigour. All that is needed is that the producer, deeply imbued with the essence of his subject, should endeavour, by a series of eliminations and restrictions, to remove from the film all unnecessary elements, to tone down others and to fuse together those he regards as the most intense and suggestive. "A work of art aims at manifesting some distinctive and essential character, and consequently some important idea, more clearly and fully than real objects do. It does this by making use of *a combination of connected parts whose mutual relations it systematically modifies*" (Taine).

In a general way, the science of human groupings and rhythmic evolutions of crowds would be better if controlled by the elementary principles which govern the construction and development of musical polyrhythms. The effects of human and æsthetic emotion that are produced by simultaneous and concurrent gestures, such as the kneeling and other movements of crowds, are nowadays mostly out of date and seem no longer to portray the sincere revelation of collective thought. At all events, producers owe it to themselves not to cultivate solely effects analogous to those of musical unisons. If at a given time the entire chorus has to make an impulsive movement, a single step forward by every member of the chorus will not give us the feeling of an advancing crowd. It wi. necessary for the last members to remain on the spot, others to take a short step, others again a longer one, and some several consecutive steps, so that the whole space may remain occupied and consequently the group may be extended.

Similarly, from the dynamic point of view, the impression of a common display of energy does not depend on the muscular expenditure of each separate individual. The *crescendo* effect may be obtained, without any increase of particular energies, by a simple contraction of the group – analogous to the contraction of a muscle – or else by an expansion which enables it to fill a larger space. In a general way all dynamic effects will be obtained by modifications of spatial relations, and all emotional effects by the interruption of symmetry. If a single person slightly rises in a kneeling group, the impression made will be stronger than if all rise simultaneously. The effect will be increased tenfold if, while the one person is rising, the other kneeling persons bow down to the ground. Just as every arm gesture has its full significance only when contrasted with some other part of the body, so collective gesture needs the contrast supplied by well-appointed conflicting attitudes. An advancing body gives a more vivid impression of advancing direction if other bodies simultaneously retire.*

Hence polyrhythm must play a very important part in the staging of crowds – not only polyrhythm in the chorus but that which counterpoints the gestures of a soloist by those of a chorus group, or contrasts continuous slow movements with quick jerky ones, links together gestures and steps in canon style, and regulates the conflict between attitudes and changes of place. In an orchestral symphonic *ensemble*, the composer offers the soloists full

* See "The Technique of Moving Plastic," p. 42.

liberty to interpret the dominant ideas of the music, but their lyrical expansion is continually being curbed and conventionalised by the necessity of respecting the limits imposed on the *ensemble*, of not disturbing the balance of the interpretation. On the screen, in all *ensemble* scenes, it is the crowd that creates the environment of the actors. These may obviously retain their individual independent action, if they try to adapt themselves to this environment imposed on them by the æsthetic and sentimental conditions of the work. On the other hand, all the grouped individualities that make up the crowd must abjure their personal mode of self-expression so as not to injure the general impression. It is for the crowd to be continually setting up relations and contrasts between the pictured life of the heroes of the drama and of normal life, as well as the fundamental rhythms of the spectators themselves.

If the film would become more one with the music, it might also abandon the more or less literary explanations on the screen, as the reading of them makes illogical pauses in the continuous movement of the pictures. To acquire æsthetic value, the arrest of movement should be effected rationally. To replace the explanations written on the screen, a singer, to very quiet orchestral accompaniment, might comment on the action in musical recitatives. Many other innovations might be attempted with the object of refining both music and scene. It would take too long to mention them all, for we have still to examine certain cases in which the music, without any sacrifice of its arrangement, may most effectively collaborate with vision.

In all gay or humorous scenes, pianist or orchestra effectively serve the actor by playing scherzos or rondos, overtures of Italian *opéra bouffe* or modern fantasias. But why should not the producers occasionally allow the music to inspire them with scenic conceptions? It would be easy for them to illustrate by human movements certain descriptive scenes to which continuous action might readily be adapted. For instance, "*L'apprenti sorcier*" of Dukas or "*Till Eulenspiegel*" of Strauss, in the realm of humour, the "*Nuit de Walpurgis*" of Mendelssohn, the "*Procession nocturne*" of Rabaud, the "*Camp de Wallenstein*" of d'Indy or the "*Horace triomphant*" of Honegger, in the realm of tragedy – these would supply the cinema with themes easy to interpret plastically and to develop throughout a continuous action.

Other musical works, such as the "Fingal's Cave" of Mendelssohn, might form a suggestive commentary on the exposition of certain landscapes wholly destitute of human presence. A mere succession of the admirable Alpine views filmed by Jacques Feyder in his masterpiece "*Visages d'Enfants*," if accompanied by the "*Poême des montagnes*" of Vincent d'Indy, would produce an effect of unity of style far different from that attained by a certain recently heard orchestral adaptation in which the humble funeral procession, sorrowfully making its way along the narrow mountain path, was accompanied by the stately music of the March from 'Tannhäuser,' while the poignant grief of a poor little countryman was expressed by one of the most thrilling passages from the supremely dramatic 'Tosca'! Suitable music may increase the value of a succession of moving scenes; but, on the other hand, a film must be of undoubted intrinsic worth to withstand the accompaniment of music totally different in style!

There is no closer association or union than that of landscape and music. The lines and contours of the former inspire and dictate the natural style and elementary development of the latter. The thousands of shades created by the play of light and wind may be transposed into the realm of sound without injuring the arrangement and evolution of the general impression. In these days of artistic conscientiousness, when certain artists frequently spend a whole year – and sometimes longer – in building up a film, it would be interesting to produce a "visio-musical" work, imposing in unity though diverse in shading, by exhibiting a landscape under the various aspects presented by the progress of the seasons – winter gradually becoming transformed into spring, the trees being decked with foliage and blossoms, the summer sun ripening the fruit, then the splendid tints of autumn, followed by the falling of the leaves and the icy clasp of winter. . . . This landscape, sometimes presented by the photographic negative which would intensify its contours, would either be stirred by slight breezes or shaken by storms, veiled in mist or fog, or slumbering beneath the caress of the noonday sun or the rising moon. Such a vision would be essentially musical, and would give the composer a splendid theme for the human symphony of the four ages of life.

In a work of this kind, the producer would not need to be altogether familiar with musical technique. Nor would it be necessary for the musician to have made a profound study of the laws of pictorial movement. Unity would be secured by a natural development of an æsthetic emotion common to both allied arts, as well as by the logical continuity of the transformations of nuances. No sooner, however, does the human element enter, infusing life and movement into the landscape, than the composer of music must learn something of the motor possibilities of the muscular system, of the laws governing the preparation and the sequence of gestures and attitudes, as well as of the various forms assumed by the rhythmic manifestations of the individual. If the power of ideas is capable of creating a suitable technique, then the knowledge of such technique will encourage the production of new ideas. These are connected with forms by powerful links. Only by the study of the human body and its powers of movement can the musician grasp the true meaning of human nature. Changes of mood and character, the rise and fall of emotion, together with the emotional impacts of man, are expressed by changes in gait and in expansiveness of physical movements, both at rest and when walking or gesticulating. These changes inevitably introduce corresponding modifications of time and dynamics into the music that attempts to express them. The duration of visual manifestations corresponds with that of sound movements, energy with energy; but division of space becomes transformed into division of time. If at any given moment of the action it is necessary that rhythms of gesture, of walking or running should synchronise with the tonal rhythms – then an acquaintance with the bodily mechanism and with musical technique should be required alike from the masters of the screen and from those of music. An amusing instance of carelessness or absence of mind is given us in a scene from "Sylvia," the charming ballet of Delibes. At a certain moment, the heroine has rapidly to cross the entire length of the stage and take refuge in the wings. "Sylvia takes flight," says the text, and, to illustrate this flight, the musician is content to have the orchestra play a simple chromatic scale in demi-semi-quavers, the duration of which might suffice for the scurrying flight of a mouse, but certainly not for that of a *ballerina*, however active.

A composer will never be able to attune his music to movements whose pace he has to emphasise, unless he can "humanise" his musical rhythms, *i.e.* feel echoing within himself the physical sensations called forth by the muscular rhythms of the actors. Indeed, it is impossible to represent a plastic rhythm musically without imagining a body in motion. To move itself, the body needs a fraction both of space and time. The beginning and the end of the movement determine the measure of time and space. Both depend on weight or gravity, *i.e.* as regards the limbs set moving by the muscles, in muscular elasticity and strength. If we determine beforehand the relations between muscular strength and the fraction of space to be traversed, we simultaneously determine the fraction of time. If we set up beforehand the relations between muscular strength and the fraction of time, we determine the fraction of space. In other words, the form of the movement results from a combination of muscular strength, the extent of the portion of space, and the duration of the fraction of time.*

If we fix in advance the relations between the portion of space and the fraction of time, then, in order to introduce proportionate movements, we must be masters of our bodily mechanisms, for lack of strength might cause the measure of space to be surpassed or the time to be shortened; on the other hand, rigidity or too great restraint would leave incomplete the fraction of space or would cause the time to be surpassed. Neither weakness nor rigidity nor inattention should modify the forms of movement; the preliminary condition of a rightly performed rhythm calls for the mastery of movements in relations of strength, space and time.

Without an acquaintance with these elementary laws, a composer will never produce the right kind of music for the screen. To spiritualise his subject, he should be thoroughly acquainted with the mysteries of muscular life, never forgetting (1) that rhythm is movement, (2) that movement is essentially physical, (3) that all movement requires space and time, (4) that physical experience forms musical consciousness, (5) that improvement of physical

* See "The Nature and Value of Rhythmic Movement," p. 11.

means results in clearness of perception, (6) that improvement of movements in time ensures the consciousness of musical rhythm, just as improvement of movements in space ensures the consciousness of plastic rhythm.

The majority of mankind have lost their instinctive rhythms; they will never recover them by the technique of the traditional choreographic art. The cinema, however, which so easily registers the movement of animals, as it does those of human beings, may powerfully contribute to a resurrection of certain natural motor impulses. Music, too, can arouse in man certain latent rhythms, through its great power of exciting, magnifying and regulating muscular dynamic forces. It is said that Charles Chaplin – and other producers – regulate some of their scenes with several characters by means of music. And they are right, for music alone is capable of regulating the relations between dynamic force and time in space. The creation of new human rhythms will be facilitated by the oppositions which material obstacles, formed by an intelligently modified space, may bring against continuous movements. Rhythm is frequently the outcome of a loss of equilibrium. Hence we see how important is the part played in stage-craft by the use of walls, columns, stairs, and variously inclined planes. The conflict between inanimate forms and living bodies inevitably produces new rhythmical expressions.

We have seen that producers have not yet thought of giving us films in which screen effects are occasionally sacrificed to give greater importance to musical effects. And *vice versa*. It is nevertheless important, if we would attain to a fundamental musico-visual art, that the orchestra of bodily movements should not constantly be using the whole of its registers. Nor will the musical orchestra,

P

in commenting on the action, be continually playing *tutti*. The composers will learn to restrict their effects, when necessary, to contrast occasionally visual with musical rhythms, and, by the alliance, the opposition, or the superposition, of tonal and pictorial movements, to built up a new polyrhythm, a counterpoint of a yet unknown kind. Here, various elements would be fused into each other, would encounter or flee from one another, overlapping or contending. To effect this, each of the allied arts must learn to value the great æsthetic and human importance of alternations of movement and pause, of vibrant resonance and of weighty silence.

Certainly we may hope for a speedy solution of the interesting problem now being debated by poets of the cinema and certain musicians, on the look-out for new artistic partnerships. Both should carefully study the common elements of their respective arts, should combine, unite and disunite them, in accordance with the natural laws of affirmation and negation, combination and conflict, struggle and consent, reinforcement and contrast. Beauty has no special form; it generally results from the harmonising of various forms. The seventh art lives so intensely that it can dispense with the aid of music, the art of sound, but once it becomes imbued with the quite peculiar sensibility of music – that art which is manifestly the most susceptible of reaching and stirring the hearts of the masses – it will have at disposal an endless diversity of means of expression, calculated to create æsthetic effects that are more fully human, emotions that are deeper and more lasting.

XIV

THE LYRIC THEATRE AND THE PUBLIC
(1922)

In any musical centre one may expect to find people of totally different artistic tendencies. There is the public of the theatre, that of symphonic concerts, and that of charity concerts, recitals of pupils and musical societies, tea, bridge, and tango concerts. Each of these brings together a number of individuals who claim to love music, and indeed do love it – since they neglect no opportunity of listening to it – though for different reasons.

Clearly there is music and music, and the æsthetic delight obtained from listening to works of "pure" music is not the same as that supplied by dramatic music. The main thing is that it should appeal to the particular sensibility of each individual and be in good taste.

The general opinion is that the principal mission of the musical theatre is to entertain. It is unnecessary here to discuss this opinion. But while it is possible for private entertainments sometimes to lack artistic character, a public entertainment may not dispense with the aid of art; indeed its social range and importance increases in proportion to the artistic element it supplies. Lyrical performances may have great influence on musical development if music is respected and placed first, if it is promulgated in accordance with the main principles of art – style, order in nuance, right proportion and sincerity of emotion.

In the case at issue it matters little, for the moment at

all events, that our opera houses give us but few classical works of first rank by Mozart, Beethoven, Grétry, Gluck, and Weber. This simply proves that their usual public neither appreciates nor demands this kind of work, and that the symphonic concert public takes little interest in the theatre. What is more important for us to know is whether the interpretation of the modern lyrical repertoire constantly testifies to a sincere desire, if not for perfection, at least for conscientious focusing. For a theatrical interpretation to be artistic, the management must regard the question of art as more important than that of gain. (It is essential that every theatre should obtain receipts sufficient for its existence – even for existence on a fairly lavish scale – it is not necessary that it should make huge profits.) All the singers must be thoroughly acquainted with their parts and their individual interpretations harmonised with a constant eye to the general effect from the vocal and scenic point of view, and from that of unity of style, both in the orchestra and on the stage. There should be perfect balance between all elements of the work, no detail should be neglected, and its main purpose and intention should be the object of profound and leisurely study, so as to leave each performer quite free at the very outset from all concern about the interpretation of his own part, and to express the fundamental emotion of the work.

Are these conditions realised on our stage? It is for the theatre-going public to reply. They know, as I do, that from the vocal point of view no exaggerated effect should be tolerated on the part of soloists, no nuance imposed by a striving after personal effect harmful to the general impression – such as ill-timed pauses and *rubati*, useless vocal outbursts, arbitrary modifications of the melodic curve, etc. The chorus should be acquainted with both the music and the main principles of the art of singing.

They should consider other things than shouting and dominating the instruments. They should sing in tune and in time, respect indications of style and nuance, listen to and harmonise with the orchestra, and know their entries sufficiently well to dispense with the necessity of keeping their eyes constantly fixed on the conductor.

As regards stage setting, the soloists will not be satisfied with wearing the costumes of the characters they represent; they should endeavour to enter completely into their personality. They will exert themselves to use other gestures than placing the hand on the heart or running the fingers through the hair, or even raising or extending both arms; they will harmonise these gestures with musical rhythms, and try to walk naturally about the stage, respecting the laws of life and motion, as well as the practices of society throughout the ages. For instance, they will not fling their cloak on to the ground immediately they enter the duke's *salon*, dash down their goblet at the end of a drinking song, leave the *prima donna* during the ritornelles of the love duet to make sure no one is watching them from behind the scenes; nor will they repeat in Italian an air that has been encored by an enthusiastic French public, nor rise from the ground with a smile to reassure a sensitive public after a painful and prolonged death struggle.

The chorists will try to march in time during the introduction of the soldiers' chorus, and not stand still in a semicircle when all the characters are on the stage. They will not indulge in a symmetrical *chassé-croisé* every twenty-four bars and repeat the same performance at the other end of the stage. The men will not manifest so strong a feeling of hatred towards the fair sex that they cannot resist the inclination to be always forming little groups of their own. The *danseuses* will avoid dancing in short white muslin drawers before a crowd of humble villagers; they will try to conceal their ambitions – after all very imperfectly realised – to soar aloft instead of moving about on solid ground like everybody else. They will dissimulate their altruistic inclination to enter into a communion of feeling with the gentlemen in the stalls, will cease to indulge in frivolous conversation during the death struggle of the tenor, and will refrain from applauding the *première danseuse* at the moment when – a "La Gioconda" smile on her lips – she attempts to cross the entire stage in a whirl of impetuous leaps expressive of the frenzied transport of the finale.

As regards orchestra and repertoire . . . But, after all, is not the critic going beyond his rights when suggesting so many *desiderata* regarding performances which three-quarters of the spectators will heartily and unreservedly applaud? The theatre – we shall be told – is instinct with tradition, and all tradition is deserving of respect. Perhaps! All the same, does not artistic progress consist precisely in reforming these traditions which seem indeed quite out of date? And have not certain theatres already set up quite new traditions more directly inspired by a desire for the natural, for style and for genuine emotion? Surely education would enable artists and public alike to distinguish between dramatic effects that spring from art and those engendered only by routine and a desire for applause.

"I should be sorry," wrote Diderot, "were my ill-interpreted remarks to cause a shadow of scorn to be cast on men of rare talent and real usefulness, in a profession I love and esteem." This profession is indeed one of the highest, and well deserving of every encouragement. That is why it is the duty of a public desirous of progress to interest itself in the stage, not only by applauding all the noble attempts which may be made, but also by condemning the faults and errors of taste which – too often, alas! – are to be found there.

* * * * *

More and more are our opera houses becoming frequented by a *bourgeois* public fond of facile pleasures and ill-prepared to listen to musical works of superior interest. As this public is devoid of a general artistic education, it can be readily understood that it does not feel annoyed by the many faults of style and good taste committed on the lyric stage.

Our schools impart to children every kind of knowledge that can be summed up in textbooks. The knowledge which more closely touches life, both individually and socially, is communicated only apart from the regular programme or curriculum through the spirit of initiative of certain conscientious teachers who take their mission in life seriously, and do their best to make their pupils not only scholars but, above all, men. Either the important role which art can and ought to play in both the inner and the outer life of society is not understood by school authorities, or else, in a spirit of indifference, they affect to know nothing about art. What wonder, then, that our young people, on leaving a school in which nothing has been done to inspire in them true musical feeling, value only the external side of lyrical performances, and can neither distinguish the various musical forms nor appreciate a truly artistic interpretation! Music is the art of projecting outwards the life of feeling by means of graduated sounds. How can we tell how expressive sounds are intended to be unless they speak in language we can understand, above all, unless they find a way quite naturally to our inner – our better – self, that which spontaneously responds to the emotion aroused by beauty, the emotion also that recreates beauty? Certainly the theatre responds to an inborn necessity of human nature.

There is not a child – even though belonging to a family for which theatre-going offers no attraction – who does not picture in his own imagination that charming game of showing forth, in fantastic and ideal dress, the various actions of his daily life and those of the adults he is in contact with. Later on, this need will remain with him – the desire to realise in gesture the creations of his imagination and the aspirations of his soul; to divide his life in such fashion that one half of him sees itself made famous and hears itself sung to by the other; the joy of collaborating with a few choice personalities in bringing out a work universally acclaimed and appreciated; the desire to undertake and carry through by physical means a common task in view of a spiritual end – all this showing how noble is the instinctive conception of the theatrical art, justifying the love for plays and also, alas, enlightening us upon the disastrous influence of a teaching that knows nothing of art and is death to everything ideal.

In point of fact, after being deeply hurt by the conventionality of interpretation in most organised theatres, the youthful spectator finally becomes accustomed to the usual methods and adapts himself to the low æsthetic level of his environment. His need for theatrical plays overcomes the repulsion of his natural convention-shocked instincts. His ignorance of superior scenic interpretations – such as are found in large towns or in a few smaller centres where the performances are liberally financed by legacies or private gifts – prevents him from imagining, and then from demanding of the lyric theatre, anything more or better than it attempts to offer. He becomes accustomed to mediocrity of conception and of stage effect; he becomes the *habitué*, indifferent to the general importance of artistic productions and exclusively interested in details of interpretation, in the comparative merits of the soloists.

How could a public totally ignorant of the simple beauty of the classic lyrical works, of the emotional or intellectual treasures contained in the dramas or operas of Monteverde, Marcello, Cimarosa, Rameau, Gluck, Mozart, Grétry, Mehul, Weber, Beethoven, and so many others – how could such a public recognise the justice of criticisms regarding our theatres made by our professional or amateur musicians, by the ordinary public of symphonic concerts? When going to listen to an opera given in the provinces, a professional musician is compelled to leave behind him those very qualities of sensibility, taste and judgment that make him a "musician." Because a public of amateurs, which has thus been robbed of musical powers, is capable of deriving pleasure from our musical entertainments, is this a reason why these should be encouraged? "Like public, like theatre," is a common saying. Unfortunately, it is only too true; but the good taste of the public is developed by education as its bad taste is developed by routine. It is the first artistic impressions that either form or deform the natural taste for the beautiful.

* * * * *

Again, do we not find that ideas of beauty and taste are being perverted in the working classes owing to the pernicious imagination of the makers of picture dramas? Have not healthy-minded people every reason to protest against certain dangerous and stupid films and to demand that the cinema should give us pictures of real artistic worth in which the splendid possibilities created by rapid changes of scene and action enable the author to effect wonders in the realm of faëry and poetry? Of course, the average cinema public would not like a cessation of the kind of picture to which they have become accustomed, just as the victim of absinth objected to the law prohibiting its sale and consumption! Still, will not generations to come feel the benefits of such a compulsory measure? Will not those who frequent cinemas be cured of their craving after sensational films? Will not the future public of a regenerated theatre, in which vocal and orchestral interpretations have been perfected by the determination of amateurs and artists to sweep away the accumulated rubbish, acquire a purer taste and a higher conception of what lyric performances should be?

In the provinces, even more than in the capital, the concert public are taking less interest in opera. They are wrong. The very fact of remaining aloof from the theatrical movement removes from them the right to exact that this movement should branch off in a new direction. Naturally, after so many shattered illusions, they dare not risk meeting with fresh disappointment! Many a time have they filled the theatre to hear and applaud some fine artistic work, but after the first performance the orchestra has relaxed its efforts and the soloists resumed their bad habits. It is not sufficient to ensure the fine interpretation of a work, efforts must still be directed towards keeping it at the level attained by strict and exceptional study. Now, this seldom happens in the provinces; too often is a work presented to the public before it is thoroughly mastered. In the largest towns, an opera is given with the aid of some famous singer from Paris or elsewhere who has not even rehearsed either with the other singers or with the orchestra. How many theatrical managers openly declare that the work they are setting up has nothing to do with art, that it is above all else a business affair and their principal desire to ensure that the takings should be sufficient to enable players, singers and orchestra to receive their pay regularly?

That is one point of view. Such being the case, however, it is the duty of the concert public to interest itself in the question of finance, to raise subventions, to attempt the impossible in order that the management may meet its financial responsibility, and so acquire the right to say something on the artistic side of the problem. Theatre *habitués*, I have already said, are accustomed to mediocre or inferior interpretations; and so we need not wonder if they do not suffer from this inadequate focusing of the question. But if, through private initiative, they are given the opportunity of hearing or seeing something superior, will they not use their powers of comparison and judgment? Is it not to their immediate interest to prefer the better to the worse? Are they bound to be like Martine in "Le Médecin malgré lui," and take pleasure in a thrashing?

For the moment there is no need to discuss the current opinion that the mission of the theatre is, above all, to entertain. Why should there not be a certain number of operettas included in the repertoire of the chief provincial theatres? After all, are not the works of Monsigny and Grétry operettas? Nevertheless, if an operetta contains carefully-written music, it should be interpreted with care; success should not depend on an adroit and pretty soprano, a clever tenor, and a picturesque comic singer. The chorus must sing correctly and take part in the action; there must be life and colour in the orchestra; the *danseuses* must show that they feel the rhythm of the music, and the light dialogue must not degenerate into coarse extravagance. What matters if the applause be lavish and the takings abundant owing to vulgar effects that readily appeal to the less cultured sections of the public? At that rate, the attendance would not fall off even if the stage were left to troupes of clowns and acrobats! An excuse for unworthy theatrical interpretations must not be found in the conviction, held by the public, that the theatre only fosters inferior manifestations of art, and that, after all, it is quite permissible occasionally to indulge in pleasures of an inferior type. Is it not amazing to find musical critics calmly tolerating from opera singers that which they would not tolerate for a moment at a concert . . . to find art critics who consider interesting attempts at plastic expression which they would despise on canvas or in marble? If we show ourselves indulgent towards the interpretation of works that are easy to stage, such as operettas, for instance, what indulgence shall we not be compelled to show towards performances of a higher type?

For it is important that each winter we should have an opportunity of listening to really artistic work of noble aim, works that have a beneficent effect on the public. Such lyrical dramas as "Orphée," "Fidelio," "Tristan" and "Pelléas et Mélisande" have the most ideal tendencies and at the same time crystallise the emotional life of an entire period; and each fresh generation should make acquaintance with them in order to understand the history of mankind. Moreover, it is of importance that they be presented carefully and conscientiously, with a strong desire to achieve true seriousness and beauty. It may be that this is a difficult problem. Indeed, musical drama affords the most varied means of expression possible to the race. In an attempt to harmonise poetry, music, dancing, painting, and the mechanical arts, it may often be found that the *ensemble* effect is compromised by inadequate particular effects. Each of these several arts should be scrupulously emphasised, so that the human personality, body and soul, may be revealed in them, and the combined influence of plastic poetry and music be used to educate the people afresh and enable them to attain to those regions of the ideal wherein all the noblest manifestations of the human mind are blended in one common harmony.

GENERAL

XV

RHYTHM AND FOLK-SONG

(1925)

Each nation has its own particular motor rhythms, expressed in everyday life by certain ways of carrying out the various tasks required by climate, environment, and social conditions.

According to the temperament, the mode of expression by language or gesture will be slow or rapid, gentle or brusque. According to the character, oratorical periods and rhythms are either precipitate or protracted, developed or condensed, slow-moving, or leaping ahead. Gestures fall in with syllables or with periods, either preceding, accompanying, or summing up the thought behind. It is by gesture, by attitude, or by vocal accent that we recognise the inhabitant of some particular town or village. Words are not accented on one side of a frontier as they are on the other. The language of the Burgundian is characterised by certain elisions due to his quick and ardent temperament, whereas the native of Franche-Comté drags or drawls each syllable. In the case of the native of the South of France, frequent inspirations call for prolonged expirations which lengthen the penultimate syllables in feminine endings. The man of the North inspires more slowly, his phrases and periods end abruptly, and his mute *e*'s are very short. The accenting of syllables varies considerably. In one district, the word 'travail' is pronounced with a long accent on the first syllable (trâvail); in another, the second syllable (travâil) ₛ accented, either long drawn out or cut off sharp. The Vaudois says: "le maître de forge"; the Parisian pronounces: "le maîtr' de forge." And these divers accents are emphasised by gestures which, in one country, are made with wrist and hand, in others with simple movements of shoulders or head, and even, in certain ultra-placid nations, solely by the eyelids.

All these modes of expression by voice or movements of the body are found idealised and 'lyricised' in the prosodic and musical rhythms of the folk-song – the direct emanation, the spontaneous and instinctive expression of the nervous and muscular, emotional and intellectual condition of the human being.

In certain folk-songs, the periods comprise two bars, in others three, four, or five bars. Short note-values, those expressed in music by quavers or semi-quavers, are grouped into fours or sixes in the songs of the South of France, whereas in the East they appear in twos or in triplets, and in the North in skips and dotted notes. There are countries, the whole of South Germany for instance, where the swing or pace of a song is kept uniform from the beginning to the end of the strophes; there are others where the *tempo* suddenly changes two or three times in the same song (cf. the gipsy songs). In certain countries, such as Spain, brilliant and well-accented rhythms are played at a regular speed, with alternate binary and ternary divisions; in some parts of France, in Russia and in Greece, the melody proceeds with very frequent changes of bar time. In Austria, the folk-songs, in valse rhythm, are performed with a continual *rubato*. These instinctive rhythms, suggested by nature and revealing a particular temperament, are also to be found in the melodic outline.

In the songs of Alpine shepherds, for example, large intervals such as fifths, sixths, octaves and tenths are necessary, so that the harmonies may resound in the great open spaces, and the vocal sound, energetically uttered and considerably prolonged, passes naturally from the middle to the high register, from the chest to the head voice. . . . In the plains, on the contrary, melodies more often proceed by conjunct degrees, without big skips.

Once the melodic outline is fixed by the environment, by conditions of space or the exigencies of temperament, it reacts in turn upon the harmonies of the songs. Sound and rhythm blend and the accompanying rudimentary harmonies change their nature; the counterpoints appear as chromatic in Scandinavia, as diatonic in Italy or Spain. Each of the elements composing the folk-song — rhythm, melody and harmony — is, in short, imperiously decreed by the soul of the people, so diverse and inapprehensible; and the predestined individuals who, from time to time, and without knowing how they do it, compose a folk-song which will be sung by successive generations when the author's name is forgotten, will have done no more than give substance to the mentality of their contemporaries, no more than realise their everyday life or express their passing emotions. Up on the mountains I once heard a young shepherd sing an air I had composed, entitled *Mon Hameau*, introducing notes of his own invention and changing the time. When I asked if he was sure that he was singing the song quite correctly, not knowing that it was my own composition he answered:

"Of course I am singing it right: my grandfather sang it in the same way as I do! . . ."

Certainly the shepherd was right in singing my song as he pleased. Was it not for him that I had composed it?

Men have always loved travelling: no matter where they go, they take with them the love of their native land and a whole treasury of songs which are permeated by the spirit of their country. Now, these typical songs which they pass on to people of another race are inevitably modified by those who adopt them after the fashion of their own particular temperament. Thus in the folklore of Brittany we find Norman songs with curious changes of rhythm, accent and melody. Certain folk-songs are sung throughout the world, in different melodic and rhythmic forms, nor is it possible definitely to formulate the original rhythm or to say in what country the melody-type was first conceived. There are many versions of the well-known air attributed to Mozart: *Ah! vous dirai-je, maman?* We find it almost everywhere in Europe, with interesting rhythmic modifications. See pp. 228, 229.

All these modifications of *tempo*, of accent and of melodic variation have come about gradually and quite naturally throughout the ages. Nowadays, however, owing to improved means of locomotion, songs rapidly cross the frontiers and are to be heard everywhere. The Parisian *chanson* is to-day sung throughout the world, and the French may be heard singing Spanish or Russian, American or English tunes, without knowing their origin. Some look upon these new acquisitions as an addition to our artistic heritage, and indeed it cannot be denied that negro rhythms have had a salutary influence upon the development of our sense of rhythm. Twenty years ago, for instance, our children were incapable of singing syncopations in the right time; and yet we now hear them quite naturally syncopating the songs of other lands. The freedom of jazz band rhythms, the extraordinary vivacity and variety of their cadences, their picturesque turns and twists, their wealth of accentuation and fanciful counter-point: all these have certainly infused new blood into musical rhythm.

This latter, though still untrammelled and living at the time of Bach, seemed since the days of Mozart to have become established in immutable traditions, lived on out-of-date metrical formulæ, and indulged in refined developments, in a symmetrical rigidity that was quite devoid of suppleness and antagonistic to all unconstrained and spontaneous movements. At the present time, owing to negro and oriental rhythms, freedom has been restored to rhythmic successions; alternating unequal bars have become natural, and arbitrary accentuations no longer astonish anyone. The old rigidity is dead, and the traditional thematic developments are replaced by variations of *tempo* and of accent. These variations arouse our attention and excite our curiosity to such a degree that we are no longer interested in the usual *stretti* and augmentations of classical music, nor in the carefully arranged dynamic nuances of romantic and neo-romantic works. Our musical fancy is greatly indebted to this novel collaboration of alien temperaments, and as a result our possibilities of musical expression are considerably increased.

Nevertheless this artistic progress has assuredly not come about without injuring our national qualities. The new acquisitions may easily check the onward march and development of our temperament and our character. At all events they risk influencing the natural evolution of the folk-song which, being the outcome of certain mental states all down the ages, should evidently not be regarded as a type fixed for all time and unlikely to encounter perceptible transformations. The changing forms of the song, however, dependent on a slow processus of experiments of every kind, cannot be radically modified from day to day under the influence of foreign sentiments. It should be noted that, while the English and the Americans are acquainted with and sing all our French songs, they none the less continue to compose songs embodying their own national characteristics, the words and music of which express wholly and irresistibly their usual mode of life and thought, whereas it cannot be denied that, for

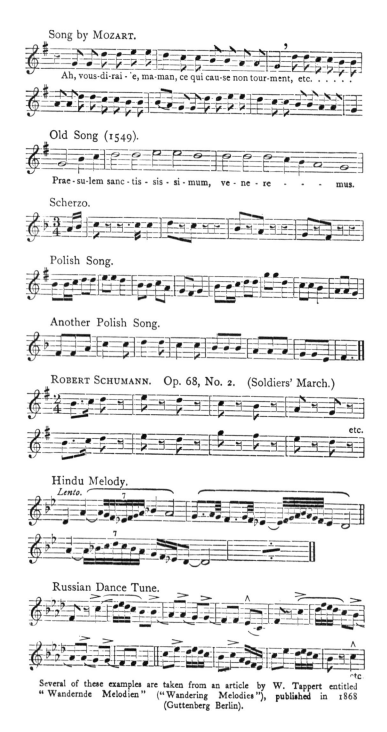

Several of these examples are taken from an article by W. Tappert entitled "Wandernde Melodien" ("Wandering Melodies"), published in 1868 (Guttenberg Berlin).

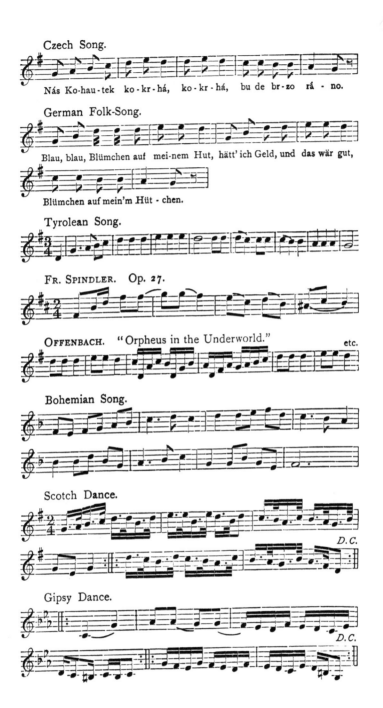

Czech Song.

Nás Ko-hau-tek ko-kr-há, ko-kr-há, bu de br-zo rá - no.

German Folk-Song.

Blau, blau, Blümchen auf mei-nem Hut, hätt' ich Geld, und das wär gut,

Blümchen auf mein'm Hüt - chen.

Tyrolean Song.

Fr. Spindler. Op. 27.

Offenbach. "Orpheus in the Underworld." etc.

Bohemian Song.

Scotch Dance.

D.C.

Gipsy Dance.

D.C.

the lyrical expression of our feelings, we are in process of adopting a mass of rhythmic forms which in no way correspond to our mental state, the nature of our feelings or the genius of our language.

As already stated, we find the accentuation of our language in the music of our folk-songs; their pace and swing, their type of phrasing and nuancing closely harmonise with the pace and swing, the direction and accentuation of our temperamental gestures. Thus in the case of the bards and troubadours, as well as of the rustic poet-singers who followed them, music and words formed one indissoluble whole. Our best folk-songs had but one author. Text and melody were composed by the same individual; the words giving birth to fitting music, the melodies governing the prosody, and the phrasing regulating the verbal periods. Now, in these days, many of our song writers readily adapt – and frequently in the most pliant and intelligent fashion – French words to melodies and rhythms of foreign origin. These adaptations may produce to some extent the impression of being natural, but they do not reveal the true genius of the language: accents are out of place, the linking together of the phrases is arbitrary. One need only 'recite' – instead of singing – a popular music-hall song of the American type, to convince oneself that our language is being travestied and that this travesty – however picturesque – discloses the elementary instincts of our race.

It will be alleged – rightly, I imagine – that music-hall songs are intended for a cosmopolitan public and do not aim at expressing our own feelings and habits. But unfortunately these songs gradually find their way among the people, both in Paris and in the provinces: they are sung in every country where French is spoken, and finally replace the simple ditties of former days, which now

gladden the hearts and lives of none but the old folk. Just
as the peasants of certain provinces are gradually laying
aside their traditional picturesque costumes and adopting
Paris fashions, so do folk-songs find themselves becoming
neglected and replaced by the airs and refrains of great
spectacular revues. The only way to remedy this disastrous state of things is for our song writers – while
continuing to write fox-trots and rhymed "ulliulla" for the
delectation of a cosmopolitan public – to devote a portion
of their time to producing words and melodies for songs
that do not disregard the natural evolution of our thoughts
and actions, and in which each of us can recognise ourselves
as we really are, in practical and emotional everyday life.

I do not mean that we ought to seek inspiration from
the folk-songs of former times, or imitate obsolete modes
of expression and repeat empty formulæ; we should rather
search deep into the soul of the nation and express that as
it really is, as we want it to continue, musically and in new
æsthetic forms – *our own* language and gestures, *our own*
spontaneous rhythmic accents, caring only to offer an
unrestrained outlet to our inmost feelings, our original
impulses. What is necessary is to sing quite simply of our
resolves and hopes, our griefs and our joys, in a way that
responds directly to all the needs of our present nature.
This nature is gradually being transformed in accordance
with the inevitable laws of evolution. Each of these transformations should find itself expressed in the songs which
our love of distinctive refinement and poetry, our direct
actions and our inmost thoughts, suggest to the poets and
musicians who represent us. Artistic internationalism
is seen in theatre and concert-room, and one would not
dream of complaining. But it is important that the simple
and ingenuous heart of a country should continue to beat
to the instinctive rhythms imposed on it by environment,

by the religious cult of ancestral deeds and thoughts, by
love of the progress still to be accomplished. And while
ear and mind rejoice in foreign songs, our tranquillity of
soul requires that we recognise and love one another, as
we sing and listen to songs which really had their birth
in our own land.

XVI

ART AND CRITICISM

(1922)

ALL artistic progress would appear to be the resultant of two forces: creation and discussion. Now, while creation inevitably incites to discussion, discussion is quite unable to produce or influence creation. The creative artist exercises a more direct influence on progress than does the critic. This does not mean that criticism is altogether ineffective: on the contrary. Indeed, it is owing to criticism that we are enabled to see how great and varied is the power of art on individuals, to compare and classify the innumerable diversities of human temperaments.

The very fact that all artistic production acts differently on individuals of opposite temperaments is proof positive how impossible it is for discussion to effect even a superficial fusion between these different types. Critics, according to their own peculiar physical disposition, see things as black or white, beautiful or ugly; they like or detest, scorn or respect works of art and interpretations of them without, as a rule, having the faintest idea that what they really admire is the expansion of their own 'self,' and that their hatred of certain artistic forms is entirely due to the fact that they are incapable of thoroughly understanding them.

Undoubtedly, it cannot be other than interesting to be able, by means of discussion, to make a physiological classification of works of art and to set up analogies between the various existing types of human sensibility.

Still, it is worth while knowing that the judgment of the most competent, conscientious and sincere critic can have no effect whatever on the development of art.

For a man of keen intellect to state periodically in writing that he likes, or does not like, some particular work of art, or some particular interpretation, is certainly interesting enough for the man himself, and also for those who feel themselves respond to the same vibrations as himself; nevertheless, the affirmation of his preferences or of his aversions has no effect whatsoever on the objects of his criticism, nor does it either increase or lessen their right to exist. Unfortunately this is not always understood by certain "regular readers" of a journal, who are but too often inclined to accept as general truths observations resulting from some particular state of mind. On the other hand, certain self-opinionated critics imagine they can advance what, in their conceit, they call truth and progress, by a constant repetition of their opinion. By dint of insistence and tenacity they may obtain temporary results, for the public are fond of being led and are willing enough to obey those with a louder voice than the rest. . . . As regards evolution, however, time is all-important; and art, the direct product of the sensibility of a people, cannot entirely change its orientation under the influence of a few isolated wills. In musical things, more particularly, judgment depends almost entirely on the receptive capacities of the organism. This is why the truly conscientious critic should repeat over and over again that the sentiments to which he gives expression are absolutely his own, and that his revelation of them can have effect only on those who feel as he does. . . . In other words, the reader of a musical criticism is receiving information, not as to the intrinsic value and the possibly universal scope of the work under discussion, but only as to the receptive powers of the critic himself.

It is quite amusing to listen to the remarks of the audience, both during and after a concert. It is even more amusing to witness their amazement the following day, when they find such contradictory appreciations appearing in their newspapers! In effect, such differences of opinion are inevitable. Every musical manifestation sets thrilling so many different fibres of our being, and gives birth to such varied emotions. A concert public brings together such opposing temperaments.

Hearing so many contradictory opinions, one wonders which is true: where genuine emotion and real wisdom are to be found. Who is right: the man who says yes or he who says no, the one who laughs or the one who weeps? And people discuss and dispute without reflecting that the music we appreciate, temperamentally, not intellectually, that to which we give ourselves body and soul, is incapable of analysis, affects individuals differently according to their own particular temperaments, and cannot be judged once for all by any human being. For the effect it produces in us depends on the way in which we respond to its influence, on the laying bare of our entire musical nature, on our efforts to become one with it and fuse it into our own soul, blending it with everything in our being that will thrill and vibrate in unison with it.

Hence, is it not the duty of all professional musicians, whom public opinion is occasionally fond of consulting, to declare whenever they have the opportunity that the praise or the blame meted out are but the revelation of their own sensitive faculties, not the affirmation of their sagacity? The development of art in no way depends on our appreciation, and the public – before paying attention to critics – will always do well to give implicit obedience to the vague warnings of their instincts, to the recommendations of their own feelings.

XVII

STYLE AND THE NEW SPIRIT
(1922)

ALL art enters upon a stage of decay when it ceases to be vivified by a new element. To keep constantly to musical forms sanctioned by time and custom is to surrender the free development of new forms: it may even be to renounce the return to old forms that have been given up and are suddenly revived by generations who feel the spirit of the past returning to life within themselves.

For everything begins over and over again: a current of intense life links the present on to the future, which itself is frequently but a resurrection of the past. Let people feel the necessity of simple homophonous forms, because they must protest against the morbid nervous state from which they suffer, and we have music reverting quite naturally to the spring of Gregorian art. Impelled by religion and a craving after purity, they may be conscious of an imperative need to blend individualities into a state of harmony that would do away with all discord: in this case we may have a revival of Palestrina. Desirous of attempting to impose a common ideal on various individualities, they may contrast harmonies with harmonies; place them above and blend them with one another; endeavour to create beauty amid a divergence of ideas and temperaments — and we find that the Stravinsky and Schönberg styles have been evolved.

The great danger, in the case of certain musical critics, is that they do not interest themselves sufficiently in the mentality of their contemporaries; do not attempt to divine what it is, in new musical manifestations, that is directly inspired by the aspirations and impulses of the people. Seldom is there escape from this danger. Beethoven's third manner, so strangely reminiscent of our present-day emotions, has on the whole not yet become classic. Modern works, evidently inspired by Beethoven in his third stage, are branded as anarchic by many of our critics, who (if they are to remain equal to their task) would need to acquire the suppleness and elasticity of mind possessed by specialists in science who, for their part, are accustomed to constant evolution, and to draw their inspiration for future progress from all the successive modifications introduced into classic attainment by new experiments.

Indeed, it is only necessary to listen to the harmonies of a fundamental fifth to understand that all sound juxtapositions, though apparently most complicated, may be justified. We need but study Oriental rhythm intelligently to understand the minds of musicians who will not remain content with processes of classic rhythm, but try to find out how much more of life, how much greater diversity, may be introduced into musical composition. It should be incumbent upon musical critics not to compare the efforts of the young moderns with the harmonic and rhythmic processes in use long ago, with which they have become familiar, but rather to explore the human mind, as well as the tendencies and intentions of innovators, taking into consideration the trend of the new spirit and analysing the nature of the impulses and aspirations awakened by a new way of living. These critics will find it a singularly difficult task to discriminate in the new forms between that which arises from a desire to astonish the natives, so to speak, and create an original style by fantastic processes – and that which is an inevitable resultant of the evolution of temperaments under the driving force of events and of the evolution of intellect in a revived social environment. This difficulty, however, is calculated to give renewed life to the critical spirit itself, so often stereotyped in set formulæ.

It is important, also, in the development of musical art, that those who "comment" should keep intellectually on the same level with those who create.

XVIII

MUSICAL ART AND THE PUBLIC
(1922)

Public taste is formed as the result of habits which people have contracted through institutions. When these are of but little interest, protests are raised in the name of art and in every town or city that claims to be a centre of art, there springs into being a whole series of small clans, each of which discusses in its own special manner the bad taste shown by such institutions. These small clans are not without their use. In the very heart of traditions regarding a style which is not above suspicion they keep alive the respect of what has been, or at all events of what should have been; they are guardians of a past, whether real or illusory; even heralds of a possible future. Unfortunately they cannot agree with one another and so have no direct influence on the artistic development of the people. The fact is they are not themselves prepared for their mission. They have not received the education suitable to them, the *clan education*. I will explain:

Artistic progress depends on education, and each personality, each group of individuals, each association of groups, needs special education. Every one of us is an echo of his environment, every artistic action is a product of the spirit of the age. Of course, genius alone can effect progress. But genius is the apanage of individuals; if it is to influence the speedy progress of the entire community it needs to be backed by groupings of talented artists. And these artists will exercise effective influence on the public only when they consent to submit to education by the strongest personalities. If every artist and association of artists looked upon artistic traditions as a precious heritage to be handed on to the young in the best possible condition and not deteriorated by use, artistic progress would be no empty word. However divergent the opinions of talented individuals, if their object is to develop public taste, they must combine in protesting against everything calculated to corrupt mankind. Once bad habits have been suppressed, it will be time to discuss the choice to be made between new habits of a different kind. Above all, scorn of everything ugly must be instilled in the mind of the public, and desire for perfection must take its place.

It is advisable to appeal to feeling, not to knowledge. Instruction is but little; education is everything. The first step along the path of regeneration is taken when we feel harassed by a desire to destroy those evil habits that constitute a barrier to progress. Nevertheless, it is clearly not sufficient to be able to destroy; it is not enough to cultivate the imagination. We must also know how to create anew. Then only is there room for instruction. Unfortunately it appears as though instruction, almost everywhere, takes precedence over education. The school attempts to instil knowledge, not to create opinions. And when some individual creates a trend of opinion the latter is seldom of general interest. Is it not indispensable that artists desirous of the progress of their country, instead of flaring abroad "art-principle rockets," should endeavour to set up "opinion-standards," to establish "æsthetical-law foundations," and to scatter among the public "beauty-idea seeds"? And to effect this, a temporary sacrifice of private opinions is needed since public taste evolves but slowly. Still, no sooner have general opinions become habitual than victory is ours, and then we have to think of propounding to the masses such modifications as they would have been unable to appreciate at the outset for want of a starting-point and through lack of conviction in the first instance.

Very many lovers of music have not sufficient *naïveté*. They go to concerts, not in order to feel musical emotions, but rather for the purpose of analysing musical processes and having the satisfaction of criticising them from a personal point of view. Instead of obeying their temperament, they listen to their reason. Instead of expanding, they contract. A musical production, however, is not a scientific thesis which can be read again and again at one's leisure and coldly analysed. Music acts on the whole of the organism like a magic force which suppresses the understanding and irresistibly takes possession of the entire being. To insist on analysing this force is to destroy its very essence. Every public body is made up both of the analytical and of the receptive. The majority of the latter are paralysed by a sort of instinctive shame created in them by age-long traditions of personal control and subjugation, of physical restraint, which may perhaps give them superior moral force, though they are thereby prevented from being frankly artists and from revealing the deep impression conveyed to the whole nature of man by the divine influence of music.

It is this feeling of shame that makes so many people prefer the stereotyped playing of works by Beethoven and Bach to freer interpretations which retain their sensorial character and restore the original impulsive life of the individual soul — this feeling, too, that causes them to prefer exhibitions of sheer virtuosity; for by public appreciation of such playing they do not compromise their inner self and yet they satisfy the scientific nature, that of every race which appreciates above all the qualities of order and style in music.

R

Still, this shame is noble in its essence and is calculated to act as a counterpoise to exaggerations in nuance, to strivings after external effects, to those cravings after pathetism which compromise the cause of music in so many superior minds. We have, on the other hand, the snobs, who manifest no shame of any kind, who testify to their swollen vanity by futile and noisy prattling, who say they are moved when they are not, who pretend to detest the very thing which has no existence so far as they are concerned, and all the time, while claiming that they hold the musical art in honour, merely practise the art of falsehood and deceit.

Between music and the public there should exist the closest collaboration. If sound reaches the human heart without being able to enter and find its abode therein, that is due to lack of musical temperament. But if, from a desire to appear sensitive, the human heart merely pretends to respond to the beneficent influence of music, then we have hypocrisy. Snobbery, while seeming to favour progress, merely causes misunderstandings, worries and annoys intelligent and sincere people, and hinders the natural development of art. It substitutes artifice for reality, contrasts imitation with nature, and replaces the genuine savour of good taste by an apparent elegance and enthusiasm.

Apart, however, from the analytical and the scientific, the shy and the snobs, there are still to be found many sensitive and thoroughly sincere individuals, enamoured of the ideal, true advocates of art and progress. Have they sufficient influence to develop the artistic sense of the people, direct their judgment, give full opportunity to their creative faculties and refine the style of their interpretations? Of course, if they could unite and protest against the evil habits acquired, if they could force the snobs to check their untimely ardour, the shy not to fear to reveal the *naïveté* of their mental state, the analytical to reconcile exigencies of style with those of temperament. . . . But the one thing to remember is that, instead of indulging in selfish enjoyment of music, they should devote themselves to spreading a taste for it in every class of society, remembering that Spencer looked upon a rational and experimental education, beginning at school, as capable of utterly changing the artistic mentality of a people within forty years.

XIX

BALANCE

The one essential law whereby we may live an harmonious life, pursue a generous idea, create or interpret works of art, or play a useful part in society and family, is that which ensures equilibrium between the forces of imagination and those of action, between will and obedience, dream and reality.

The necessity for this equilibrium is seen in every detail of our social, practical or emotional life. Both elementary and advanced instruction ought to insist upon a just balancing of the mental and the physical powers. Is not bodily fatigue compensated by mental freedom, and brain fatigue by the collaboration of the muscular system, by the unimpeded circulation of the nerve currents and by the joy that results from intelligent work done under the right conditions.

There must be set up a balance between the activity which the child applies to his lessons and the work he is called upon to do at home. Whatever is not immediately understood in class should be gone over in the silence of his own room where the mind has time to examine the question from every angle, and where solitude, after the animation of a lesson in class, conduces to action of another kind, which is more direct and definite, as well as more personal. Has not the teacher also to maintain balance in the relations between pupils, relations so often dependent upon chance, and therefore badly chosen? Discreet intervention on his part would be advisable to ensure harmony in groupings made up of such varied temperaments.

Since teachers and taught spend two-thirds of the day together, there ought surely to be established harmonious and sympathetic relations between them, even though certain sacrifices be called for on both sides.

It is evident that private study becomes easier for the child if he feels that he has none but well-disposed companions around him working with like earnestness for a common end, whom he can consult or aid.

Is it not necessary to show the child that, if he would come into close and more direct contact with his comrades, he is expected to make certain sacrifices of time and *amour-propre*?

There will also have to be much sacrifice on the part of those who enter upon the career of the teacher, a career which most imperiously calls for perfect equilibrium between one's own personal tendencies and those necessitated by teaching between the reason and the heart, between individual sympathies and the collective sympathy due to the community. The teacher has continually to be striking a balance between his interest in some particular pupil and the general interest he is bound to show for the whole class, between his instinctive desire to be indulgent and the necessity of occasionally being strict; or, on the other hand, between his individual resentments and a general spirit of impartiality and justice. Here we have very often a veritable duel between temperament and character. In class, the teacher desires to make progress, but it is necessary for the general good to sacrifice interest to security, to recapitulate instead of venturing upon new territory. He may have prepared quite a good and original lesson; and then be unable to give it because something warns him that the pupils are not yet sufficiently advanced to understand it. He is tired and would like his lesson to follow the broad and easy path, when suddenly questions asked by pupils compel him to lash himself into a condition to supply the right answer or to plan out some future lesson. . . .

There has also to be set up equilibrium between a teacher's duties – first to his pupils, next to the school, and lastly to the parents. The confidence of the children is necessary, but that of the mothers is equally so, both as regards himself and as regards the quality of his teaching. And the one confidence is so different from the other that he is frequently obliged to give proof of the utmost sagacity if the situation is to be met, conscientiously gauging the interests of each side, reflecting on the consequences of hasty solutions, and doing everything possible to effect the compromise which is so often necessary between the life of the child in school and his submission to the teacher, between the life of the child at home and his submission to family duties.

But the most difficult task is to harmonise our own faculties, to refrain from paying special attention to certain intellectual needs at the expense of the general education, to hold certain ambitions in check, to rid ourselves of certain fears and to attach the same interest to various kinds of studies, all of which are necessary for the expansion of the personality. Is it not most important that we should feel perfectly balanced in ourselves, since life compels us to set up an equilibrium, both stable and flexible, between our individuality and society? Then let heart and mind, soul and body, live that same harmonious life which controls the muscular and nervous systems in the course of our physiological studies.

A teacher's career is the finest of all; nevertheless, it exacts of every one of us a constant balance between our reasoning faculties and our spontaneous instincts. We have to weigh the pros and the cons, to harmonise the present, the past and the future, to dispense with useless thoughts and gestures, to be both serious and light-hearted, strict and lenient, imaginative and constructive, artists and artisans, doers and dreamers, teachers and pupils, ever bent on establishing equilibrium between the progress we should call forth in others and that which we should ourselves realise for the joy and security of future generations.

I regret that music in schools is often taught in too arbitrary and academical a fashion; it has no close connection with school life at all. Indeed, is it not true that, speaking generally, at school the child is not shown life as it is, he is not taught to understand even the humblest duties of life? Certain counsels given when he is very young have enormous influence upon his conduct.

If the child were taught the simple laws of equilibrium and shown how easy it is to strike an harmonious balance between actions that are often contradictory, life would be made much easier both for himself and for all around him.

Every act should find its compensation in another act.

When a mother slaps her child for being disobedient, she afterwards kisses him and says: "Now that I have punished you, I may kiss you, and we are quits" (balance of revengeful contraction and satisfied decontraction). Publicly a man treats his fellow-citizen as a scoundrel because the latter expresses political opinions opposed to his own; then, as they leave the building, he pats him on the shoulder, with the words: "You know, old man, this makes no difference to our friendship" (balance of civic reflex and individual reflex).

This search after equilibrium in everyday life should prevent the teacher from exacting of his pupils any rigid – and therefore contracted – bodily attitude, when he is calling for close attention and requiring of them a "cerebral contraction." A pupil called upon to reflect should be in a relaxed condition. The attempt to find equilibrium gradually leads teachers to vary their methods, to introduce recreation even during the hour's lesson, to relax effort whenever such a course seems necessary, to have a song sung during the geography lesson, or to ask some question in mathematics or history between two verses of a song. The natural development of their inventive faculties is as essential to the progress of children as that of their powers of imitation and mechanical repetition.

The duties of daily life are as important as those connected with school. Memorising and reasoning need to be counterbalanced by cultivating imaginative conceptions and educating the reflexes of thought. Actions, reactions and analysis: these are the elements to be combined, associated and dissociated. School hours should not be exclusively occupied by the consideration of problems foreign even to the child's personality. There should be a continual effort to set up a stable equilibrium between the teacher's adult mentality and that of his school days. He should always try to instil into the child's mind that he is as keenly interested in him when he has returned home or is playing with his schoolfellows as when he sees him, book in hand, diligently poring over his lesson. There should be no such thing as two distinct lives, that of the school and that of the family, resulting in the teacher giving him special homework that is out of harmony with his home life. On the other hand, it is indispensable that parents should interest themselves in school life, and not compete with it. What a good thing for the natural and regular development of teaching would be a university course for parents! How easy it would make the teacher's task if mothers actively collaborated with him and unobtrusively supported his teaching! It is just when parents reach the age to understand clearly what education is that they find themselves deprived of something indispensable to instruction: collaboration with the school itself. On the other hand, might not unmarried teachers benefit by special instruction enabling them to understand the close relations which should be set up between school and family life? They could then, from actual experience, call upon their pupils for those sacrifices of *amour-propre* and individual freedom necessitated by social life. They would also understand, better than do most of them, the effect of music upon the psycho-physical equilibrium of children, upon the development of their spontaneity and sensibility, the subordination of their own particular instincts to those of a social nature which are called for by that group-life so fully realised in class singing. A school in which the musical education is relegated to a second place, and choral singing does not form an integral part of the curriculum, is deliberately depriving itself of all opportunity to raise the feelings of the children to a higher plane, to enable them to soar above a material world, to follow after an ideal, to become one with everything that contributes to the formation of good taste and constitutes a natural and unconscious pre-paration – as well as a sure one – for artistic inspiration and enjoyment.

XX

CONTRADICTIONS AND INCONSISTENCIES
(1922)

THERE is no work of art that is more difficult to criticise objectively than music. If we read a number of musical criticisms by the same person, in a single volume, we find contradictions or inconsistencies on almost every page.

The musical taste – if the idealists will pardon me – is akin to the culinary taste, in the strictest and the least poetical manner. In spite of education, of temperamental unity and the will to submit to a régime, the stomach is a slave to certain immoderate appetites, as it is to certain dislikes. The musical ear also, even though guided by a very sure judgment and controlled by a firm determination to be fair and just in classing and appraising certain works, will never be able to appreciate all kinds of music. How frequently we experience the same tastes as some musician of our acquaintance, love the same schools, the same authors, the same *virtuosi*, and yet find ourselves quite opposed to him as regards a certain personality, a certain work, even a certain part of a work. The analytical faculties often play but a secondary part in musical judgment. It continually happens that a critic – after formulating *ex cathedra* these various laws of balance and construction, judgment, administration and sensibility whose *ensemble* ensures the success of a sonata or a symphony – proclaims his disdain for a composition which nevertheless obeys all these laws and so possesses the qualities which justify it in being regarded as a masterpiece. . . .

While the personal musical taste irresistibly influences the judgment of the critic, it often happens that this very taste is influenced by certain circumstances of time, place and atmosphere, as well as by the general state of the organism, at a time when it is imagined that appeal is being made to the auditive faculties alone. A particular musician would often feel pleasure in a work, did he not at the very time he is listening to it suffer from some nervous affection or from depression caused by something that has nothing to do with music. He will feel bored at listening to a certain piece because it does not respond to his mental state *at the time*, or perhaps because it is signed by a musician whose works are antipathetic to him or is played by a virtuoso of an opposite school, because he has just been practising it himself, and automatically gives it a different interpretation, or finally just because he got out of bed on the wrong side, as people say, and so everything in art and nature just then seems devoid of grace and charm, light and joy, emotion and beauty.

These contradictions and inconsistencies are due to the extreme sensibility peculiar to musicians and must be judged with kindly indulgence. But what are we to think of those caused solely by the absence of discernment and deduction, of analysis and the instinct of comparison, which should form the indispensable stock-in-trade of the critic? Even the most apparently emancipated critics are held in thrall by the invisible chains of routine; the various modes of musical realisation are not always governed by the general laws of the processes of expression, the characteristic presentation of emotions and the refining of thought, but too frequently by a number of special and self-contradictory traditions. Some day I intend to inquire more minutely into this subject – one that is seldom touched upon; for the moment, I will state a few of

the more usual contradictions in the form of questions
devoid of apparent order or logical connection with one
another.

How is it that the *rubato* style adopted by most pianists
is generally regarded as a favourable proof of sensibility,
whereas it would not be tolerated for a moment in an
orchestral performance? Is the playing out of time and
over-emphasising the left-hand *arpeggios* in a Chopin
nocturne more excusable than a disorderly or extravagant
performance of viola and 'cello *arpeggios* in the moving
Andante con moto (A flat) of Beethoven's Twelfth Quartet
(1st part)? Can there be two ways of apprehending time
and style, the first appealing to the orchestra in one direction and the second to the piano in another? We may
take for granted that this is so, for musicians would
certainly not tolerate on the part of a conductor the disorderly *accelerando*, the languishing *allargando*, the hic-
cough-like phrasings which in pianoforte performances
do not disturb them at all. Anyone singing a piece by
Schumann or Fauré in the jolting spasmodic fashion of
many celebrated pianists would be forced to retire crest-
fallen before the scorn of a justly outraged audience.
Why is a singer blamed for a nasal accent whereas no
fault is found with an oboist, a 'cellist, or a string quartet
using the mute? . . . How is it that we do not tolerate
the *tremolando* of a human voice and yet admire it in a
violinist or in the tremulant or bourdon stops of the organ?
. . . Would a symphonic orchestration that gave the same
impression of sonority and timbre as the full swell of the
organ be regarded as artistic?

The exaggerated pauses of the Italian singer are no
longer applauded by any but a public that craves after
effects in bad taste. Why are refined musicians not
shocked when they hear the improvisations of most

organists brought to a triumphant conclusion in a crashing intoxication of sound? Why are 'vocalises' condemned in present-day opera and admired in Mozart and Handel? Why are effects of virtuosity looked upon as obsolete and technical exercises lacking in artistic value in modern piano works (Chopin studies and Liszt and Saint-Saëns concertos), whereas they are tolerated in an *allegro* of Scarlatti, the variations of Rameau, the *gigues* of Graun or Frescobaldi . . . even in the concertos of Beethoven?

It is generally regarded as an unpardonable sin for a virtuoso to play a prelude for piano or organ without the succeeding fugue, or a fugue without the prelude – or even to detach some particular number from a suite and play it separately. Very well. But why is it considered perfectly natural for an orchestra to perform at a concert the 'Overture of Leonora' or of the 'Nozze di Figaro,' the Prelude of 'Tristan' (even the Introduction of the Third Act with the *cor anglais* solo) without following them up with the act for which it is their mission to prepare the listener? Why are isolated fragments from the ballets of Rameau and Gluck generally given without a voice being raised to protest against such mutilation?

Critics easily explain away these contradictions and many others by quibbles or ingenious artifices of mental transposition, by confronting instrumental techniques and styles. There is, however, a vast domain in which the inconsistent judgments of the most reputed artists become quite inexplicable. This is the domain of such allied arts as: music and verbal expression, music and decoration, music and bodily movements, music and light. On this branch of the subject we will consider a few general questions of elementary import.

How comes it that so many painters, possessed of the most sensitive and penetrating vision, can tolerate in the theatre the vivid glare of light projections, the deception created by footlights?

How can sculptors, whose talent owes its entire effect to their ability to detect the secrets of the art of movement and of every phase of the balance and energy of the body, appear at a spectacle dealing with plastic art, without manifesting the faintest repulsion at the lack of naturalness, of diversity and of expression in the gestures or attitudes of actors or dancers, at the conventionality of their movements, the paucity of their physical means of expression and the exaggeration of their methods?

Why is it that specialists in verbal rhythm are never shocked by the faults in prosody of lines set to music? And lovers of fidelity to thought and expression, psychologists, philosophers, simple observers of life in its various emotive manifestations, put up with the usual conventional theatrical situations, the pomposity of dramatic processes, the grandiloquent tirades, and the *cabotinage* of stage heroics?

Concerning musicians especially, how can the same critics – uncompromising as regards purity of phrasing, rhythm and delicacy of shading – feel no concern whatsoever at the absence of any relationship between the gestures of dramatic singers and dancers and the musical phrases they are endeavouring to express, at their lack of bodily sensibility and their constant assaults on rhythm, and even time, on style, on musical fidelity or honesty, in a word, on 'music' itself? A pianist will be blamed for playing an organ piece transcribed for the piano, and *vice versa*, whereas applause is bestowed on the approximative scenic realisations of a Schumann 'Carnival' or of symphonic poems by Rimsky-Korsakov, D'Indy, Dukas, or Debussy.

Let an artist attempt to offer the public means of dramatic expression inspired by a profound and minute study of the laws of artistic association, by the concordance between gesture and music, gesture and word, groups of attitudes, light and space . . . and there will be found but few instinctively capable of keeping pace with these new conceptions. In the theatre, special traditions have perverted and distorted fidelity to truth both physical, poetical, musical, and human.

Respect for the qualities of simplicity and expression, order, construction, appreciation, sacrifice and balance, which every artist regards it as a duty to observe himself and to impose on others in his own particular branch of art, is trampled under foot by three-quarters of the specialists who have to judge of a work that brings together different arts. The reason of this singular attitude is to be sought in the ignorance of most specialists concerning the special art of synthesising the various means of artistic expression. The present-day culture of many artists is incomplete; their ignorance is flagrant. It is the 'human' factor that is lacking.

No evolution at all is possible without the aid of conscious or unconscious education, either imposed by the events of life or created by the human will.

XXI

WAITING FOR REFORMS
(1922)

"How downhearted you look to-day, Mr. Everyman! Can it be that you, so fervent a lover of music, have had to go through the anguish and torture of listening to something altogether ear-splitting and discordant?"

"Well, I confess I do feel somewhat exasperated when I find in all our musical periodicals articles dealing with the necessity of reforming musical instruction. For some time past our critics have been able to talk of nothing but reform! Who could help thinking that the musical art is in a state of decadence? Whereas you know quite well that there has never been so much music in Paris as since the Treaty of Versailles! Have we not first-class schools of music?"

"Assuredly."

"Famous music teachers and pupils in great numbers, unique orchestras and the best of conductors?"

"Undoubtedly."

"Are not our State-subventioned lyric theatres, as they have always been, perfectly well adapted to the finest interpretations?"

"They are."

"Are we not indebted to private initiative for periodical performances and auditions of works both new and old, vocal and instrumental, interpreted by the most gifted artists?"

"Such initiative merits our deep gratitude."

"In the provinces are there fewer singing classes and choral societies than before the war, fewer dramatic clubs, etc.? No, I really do not believe that there is any country so well provided as our own with artistic associations of every kind. Our artistic sensibility is everywhere in evidence; it is even a matter of no small difficulty to direct it along the right channels, so rich and impetuous are its springs. Certainly there is scarcely to be found a single individual who, on attaining to a certain position in society, is not a member of at least two or three musical, artistic or literary committees."

"I do not deny the existence of all these artistic clubs, nor the innumerable musical resources at the disposal of the nation."

"Well?"

"Well, Mr. Everyman, all I can do is to repeat once more that our artistic progress does not depend on the greater or less number of educational means placed at the disposal of the people by private initiative, but rather on the way in which these various means may, in an organised fashion, develop individually, in the first place, and then collectively those whose ideas represent the spirit of our race. More than any other art, music has the power to unite individuals, to instil in them a univeral spirit of union and combination, and to create within the very heart of this organised society a focus of living enthusiasm and emotional activity.

"Up to the present, however, music has been a privileged art, reserved for a minority of aristocrats in feeling and thought, an art whose manifestations its followers attempt to direct along the lines of a purely sensorial specialisation which aims solely at the enjoyment of the organs of hearing. Since, however, a grievous and prolonged war has put all nations in mourning, it appears as though it has become the role of music to rise far above that of a 'prince's pastime,' conferred on it by Rameau and *tutti quanti.* The new role it is called upon to fill is that of 'leader of men and nations.' Its influence consists in revealing man to himself, instilling into him a powerful and subtle magnetic influence, and then inspiring in him an irresistible desire to join in communion and fellowship with all his fellow-creatures who are alike conscious of lofty and noble human feelings, distributed and expanded by the magic of sound and rhythm."

"You are quite right. Was it not Diderot who said, 'La musique est l'art social par excellence'? We all agree on this, and our innumerable musical schools and societies testify to the rational enthusiasm of our intellectual classes."

"They certainly testify to the fact that there is a great deal of goodwill, Mr. Everyman, but they do not put music in a position to fill that ideal role we insist on assigning to it. Oh, of course, it is of the utmost importance that in every school and society there should spring up and manifest itself a spirit which has been breathed into their disciples by the talented persons who direct them. In the course of the ages, human society has never developed by any other means than the far-sighted will and determination of the elect few. It is not enough, however, that any considerable number of our artistic associations should each possess a collective temperament made up of artistic acumen, of the will to progress, and of power trained in the externalisation of thought. The one thing of importance is that each of these 'group spirits' should enter into communication with 'group spirits' of another essence, and that between all these agglomerations of individuals there should spring up mutual love to inspire them with strength and life."

"All the same, we know that from the earliest times men have never agreed or been of one mind. And in the special domain of art is it not an acknowledged fact that each specially gifted individual possesses a temperament different from that of the rest, and that it is this very difference that assigns to him a place apart in the history of progress?"

"It is indeed thus – very fortunately for progress – that things have always happened! But whereas each of us daily recognises that the fact of imparting to friends or strangers our own special feelings and thoughts, at once enables us to examine these feelings and thoughts from another angle, in a clearer and more general fashion and under a more universal aspect, how could we help expecting from the exchange of group ideas so manifestly favourable a result? Each of our schools of music lives its own life: each of our great choral societies does the same. This too may be said as regards the numberless artistic groupings in the provinces. It is thus evident that the country, as a musical whole, is conscious that there is, thrilling within its bosom, a vast number of lives. But does this in itself give proof of a truly organised life? Each association goes its own way; it cannot find time either to inquire into or become inspired with the desires of its neighbours. Each follows its own particular path, whether narrow or broad; each draws upon its own supply of ideas, whether small or large. All these scattered flames do not keep alive a common centre of heat and light."

"So you would like the committees of our associations and societies, at the beginning of each season, to group together for the purpose of exchanging ideas and plans and evolving a collective programme of study and entertainment?"

"That is just what many artists desire."

"My dear fellow, do you imagine that all this would come about without dispute and controversy?"

"Most likely not; still, we should learn to know each

other: a consummation devoutly to be wished! All these interesting little clans into which our artistic life is split up and divided are not only ignorant of one another but actually avoid opportunities of becoming acquainted. Let them but group together and – at once – a new life will open out before them. The spirit of self-respect and of emulation, curiosity regarding differences of ideas, will act as a spur to the various temperaments. Thus we shall see the awakening of the state of mind peculiar to associations of people animated by the same love of the ideal, that state of mind in which the intentions of others are not suspected merely because they seem strange or foreign. Nothing but public discussion is capable of proving the sincerity of those who introduce new ideas into the world. As soon as our 'clans' consent to meet together for the elaboration of a general education and artistic programme, whatever be the result of their deliberations, each of them will assuredly return home with greater esteem for the intentions of the others and confirmed in its own fundamental ideas by reason of the open discussion to which these will have been subjected."

"And yet every bank acts on its own initiative, our charity organisations and provident societies do not dream of combining, our coal industry and our provision trade. . . ."

"Mr. Everyman, we are speaking of sentiment, not of business; more especially are we speaking of musical feeling. Were music suited for nothing else than to provide a little consolation for isolated souls, we should assuredly never dream of urging human beings to meet together for the purpose of basing on it alone their common hopes. But it is musical rhythm that has united men in groups ever since the world began. The early Christians assembled for religious dancing and the singing of hymns expressive of the solemn fervour of their devotions. And our modern theatrical art was born of the initial attempts at the groupings of enthusiastic crowds. The immediate result – in every canton – of the popular Swiss 'Festspiels' has been to silence individual malice and ill-will, and to promote union among all who are enamoured of the same patriotic or religious ideal. A religion founded on mutual love cannot do other than encourage a cult of beauty and truth, under whatever form it appears."

"And so you dream of democratising music?"

"I dream only of restoring it to its natural functions, which are social in their essence. Surely one so worthy as yourself, Mr. Everyman, cannot but acknowledge that I am right!"

"Yes, yes, of course. . . . All the same, granting that there is something in your ideas (I shall have to make inquiries on the matter), don't you think – we have so many other good objects to work for – that we might yet wait a little longer before attempting to realise these projects of yours? It seems to me we have so many other irons in the fire just now!"

"Then let us combine for the 'waiting'!"

INDEX